Candida Albicans

"An excellent book for understanding and fighting against candida-related health problems. A clearly explained, simple to follow, and detailed anticandida program."

CHRISTOPHER VASEY, N.D., AUTHOR OF
THE ACID–ALKALINE DIET FOR OPTIMUM HEALTH
AND *NATURAL REMEDIES FOR INFLAMMATION*

Candida Albicans

Natural Remedies for Yeast Infection

A 10-Point Plan

Leon Chaitow, D.O., N.D.

Healing Arts Press
Rochester, Vermont • Toronto, Canada

Healing Arts Press
One Park Street
Rochester, Vermont 05767
www.HealingArtsPress.com

Healing Arts Press is a division of Inner Traditions International

First edition published in 1985 by Thorsons Publishing Group, London;
  reprinted in 1987 by Thorsons Publishing, Inc.
Second edition published in 1988 by Healing Arts Press
Third revised and expanded edition published in 1998 by Healing Arts Press
Fourth revised and updated edition published in 2016 by Healing Arts Press

*Note to the reader: This book is intended as an informational guide. The
remedies, approaches, and techniques described herein are meant to supplement,
and not to be a substitute for, professional medical care or treatment. They should
not be used to treat a serious ailment without prior consultation with a qualified
health care professional.*

Library of Congress Cataloging-in-Publication Data
Names: Chaitow, Leon.
Title: Candida albicans : natural remedies for yeast infection : a 10-point plan
  / Leon Chaitow, D.O., N.D.
Description: Fourth edition. | Rochester, Vermont : Healing Arts Press,
  [2016] | Previous edition: Candida albicans : could yeast be your problem?
  (Rochester, Vt. : Healing Arts Press, 1998). | Includes bibliographical
  references and index.
Identifiers: LCCN 2016013120 (print) | LCCN 2016015975 (e-book) |
  ISBN 9781620555811 (pbk.) | ISBN 9781620555828 (e-book)
Subjects: LCSH: Candidiasis—Popular works. | Candida albicans—Popular
  works.
Classification: LCC RC123.C3 C48 2016 (print) | LCC RC123.C3 (e-book) |
  DDC 616.9/693—dc23
LC record available at https://lccn.loc.gov/2016013120

Printed and bound in the United States by Versa Press, Inc.

10 9 8 7 6 5 4 3 2 1

Text design and layout by Virginia Scott Bowman
This book was typeset in Garamond Premier Pro and Avenir with Novarese
used as the display typeface

To send correspondence to the author of this book, mail a first-class letter to
the author c/o Inner Traditions • Bear & Company, One Park Street, Rochester,
VT 05767, and we will forward the communication, or contact the author
directly at **www.leonchaitow.com** or at **leonchaitow1@mac.com**. *Please note:*
No health advice can be offered via this medium.

Contents

Acknowledgments

The pioneering research of Dr. C. Orion Truss in the uncovering of candida's involvement in a wide range of diseases and conditions deserves recognition; I respectfully dedicate this book to him. Others who have made major contributions to this knowledge, to whom I owe my gratitude, include Dr. William G. Crook and Dr. Jeffrey Bland. In this book I have quoted from all three of these respected scientists, and on behalf of all those who will benefit from their original work I thank them. The books of Dr. Truss and Dr. Crook (*The Missing Diagnosis* and *The Yeast Connection,* respectively) are worthy of study by anyone who wishes to have a deeper knowledge of this subject.

CHAPTER 1

Candida Yeast and Common Health Problems

Since the mid-1980s it has become clear that an increasing number of common health problems, both physical and mental, might have something in common—namely, the spread in the body of a yeast that lives in each and every one of us. Its name is *Candida albicans*—candida for short.

Since the first edition of this book was published in 1985, a major part of my practice has involved people with candida overgrowth and its associated health problems, which commonly include symptoms of chronic fatigue, irritable bowel syndrome (IBS), allergies, and fibromyalgia. The worldwide scale of this problem has become increasingly apparent to me as a result of the stream of letters I have received over the years from readers of this book. Many of the people who have written to me have said that this book changed their lives; they tell heartbreaking stories of desperate health situations that have been positively transformed (although not overnight) by the application of the principles detailed in this book.

While receiving such letters is truly gratifying, the real credit should go to the pioneers of research into this subject, namely the American physician C. Orion Truss, who was the assistant chief of medicine at the U.S. Air Force Hospital at

Maxwell Field, Alabama, who made his life's work the study of candida. This American clinician was the first to introduce the world to a yeast fungus in the gut that he said was responsible for a vast range of human ailments. Since then, the name of that yeast, *Candida albicans,* has become a watchword for the many millions of people who have sought unorthodox answers when conventional medicine has failed them. Dr. Truss has written his own story of his research, and the whole story of candida, in his book *The Missing Diagnosis.*

It was Dr. Truss who first noticed what no one else seemed able to see, although it was staring them right in the face. Because the fungus candida is present in all people from the first few months of life on, it tends to be overlooked by doctors seeking the causes of particular diseases or conditions. Since it is present in everyone, it seems that many of these doctors think that it could not possibly be causing any of a wide range of symptoms, including muscular pain, extreme fatigue, allergies, irritable bowel, and brain fog—all symptoms of yeast overgrowth. This way of thinking has blocked the medical establishment's focus on candida, except in rare instances in which it spreads to such an extent as to become life-threatening, something that may occur in people whose defense mechanism—the immune system—has become weakened by disease or drugs (whether used in therapy or abused). This may help us understand why a great many people suffer from a less pronounced spread of candida, which, although usually not severe enough to endanger life, is certainly sufficient to produce or aggravate a wide range of often debilitating symptoms. These include:

- depression
- anxiety

- unnatural irritability
- digestive symptoms such as diarrhea, constipation, bloating, and heartburn
- extreme fatigue and a sense of hopelessness
- an inability to concentrate, i.e., "brain fog"
- allergies
- acne
- migraine headache
- widespread muscular pain
- cystitis
- vaginitis
- thrush*
- menstrual problems and premenstrual syndrome

Understanding the way in which such a wide range of symptoms can result from the effects of a yeast that lives in all of us demands that we appreciate those factors that encourage the spread of this yeast.

In most people there is an uneasy truce between the body and the yeasts that live in it. Over many thousands of years, a balance has been struck. Yeast can live, and thrive, and present no problems to the body, as long as it confines itself to local areas such as the digestive tract. Should it spread beyond these sites, various checks and balances help to control it. The body's immune system, including the white blood cells, can attack and destroy the yeast. Also assisting in yeast control

---

*Note that the word *thrush* is commonly used to describe all yeast/candida infections, such as those affecting the mouth and the vagina, as well as those causing "diaper rash" in infants, although it more specifically describes a yeast infection characterized by white patches on the membranes of these areas.

are the "friendly" bacteria that live in and on us in return for services they provide. There are also actual physical barriers, such as the mucous lining of the digestive tract, which, when in a good state of health, prevents intrusion by yeast or any other undesirable elements. All mucous membranes contain further protective substances that can destroy invading particles of yeast.

SO WHY DOES CANDIDA SPREAD?

At this stage we should simply recognize that the body possesses an efficient defense capability for dealing with toxins, bacteria, and yeast, should any of them intrude into areas in which they present a danger. But problems arise when, because of one of a variety of causes, our ability to defend against candida weakens. As long as yeast remains in territories where it does not represent a threat to health, it is tolerated. If, however, for whatever reason, immune function is compromised as a result of antibiotic or steroid medication being used excessively, so weakening the normal flora that helps control yeast activity; and/or if dietary intake of sugars is excessive, so "feeding" yeast, this results in the multiplication of yeast cells, that then colonize areas of the body normally out of bounds. And this is precisely the combination of factors that has been identified as having become so widespread in Western society over the past fifty years.

The Problem of Antibiotic Use

The introduction of broad-spectrum antibiotics, the widespread use of the contraceptive pill, and the proliferation of steroid medications have all played a part in candida's growth.

Add to this the increase in the use of sugar and sugar-rich foods, and now you have a situation in which the yeast has just the sustenance it loves. It is this unfortunate combination of factors that is the root cause of a problem for so many people.

In the early 1990s, in a series of Fibromyalgia Network Newsletters, a San Francisco–based physician, Carol Jessop, summarized the range of yeast-related conditions she identified in over a thousand of her patients with chronic fatigue syndrome and/or fibromyalgia. Among the most common symptoms reported by her patients were: chronic fatigue (100 percent), cold extremities (100 percent), impaired memory (100 percent), frequent urination (95 percent), depression (94 percent), sleep disorder (94 percent), and muscle aches (68 percent). Dr. Jessop reported the presence of yeast infections in 87 percent of these patients. Of the 880 patients specifically tested for yeast overgrowth, 82 percent had significant levels of yeast in their stool samples, and a further 30 percent had parasites in these samples.

Dr. Jessop also investigated the symptoms these patients had experienced before their conditions became chronic: irritable bowel symptoms (89 percent); recurrent childhood ear, nose, and throat infections (89 percent); gas and bloating (80 percent); endometriosis (65 percent); constipation (58 percent); heartburn (40 percent); recurrent sinusitis (40 percent); and recurrent bronchitis (30 percent). Notably, most of these infections had been treated with course after course of antibiotics—of which the connection to yeast overgrowth and digestive distress will become clear in later chapters of this book.

It is important to understand that the conditions listed

above are certainly not always the result of candida infection. It is, however, true that all of these conditions can be partly or entirely a result of candidiasis. And so it is the view of those practitioners who are now aware of the possibility of candida's involvement in health problems of this sort that when a combination of these symptoms appears in a person with no other apparent causes, then candida should be the prime suspect.

In many cases, candida only proliferates when there is an existing pathology, such as inflammatory bowel disease (including colitis, Crohn's disease, and gastric and duodenal ulcer). In such cases it has been shown that the presence of the colonizing yeast aggravates the condition as well as delays the healing process, particularly after the use of antibiotics. It is suggested by researchers that antibiotic treatment, as well as inflammation, disturbs the balance of normal, "friendly" resident bacteria, allowing candida to colonize the gut.

TESTING FOR CANDIDA

Unlike most infections and infestations, it is difficult to test accurately for the presence of candida to prove or disprove its active presence. This is because, as has already been stated, candida is present to some extent in all of us, which makes looking for it as pointless as searching for the proverbial needle in a haystack. We know it is present, but to what extent? Candida can be cultured in many people's blood, and it is so common in stool cultures that it is usually ignored by microbiologists when they do come across it, unless it is present in significant amounts.

Medical researchers have highlighted the difficulty of assessing, purely from tests, whether candida is active, even when it is in an advanced stage of overgrowth. In one group of forty-eight patients with acute myeloid leukemia, there was such widespread candida in the lungs and other organs that "entire microscopic fields were filled with mycelia," and yet the diagnosis could have been assumed from signs without waiting for the time-consuming proof positive from the laboratory. Half of these patients died from candidiasis, and the doctors asserted that had they been able to attack the yeast aggressively at an earlier time, the tragedy might have been averted.

Among the ways to determine whether candida is present:

- Fecal culturing of candida can be helpful in identifying specific strains of yeast as well as their quantities, although researchers report that this gives 25 percent false negatives. That is, in 25 percent of cases when a stool analysis reports that a person does not have a candida overgrowth, there may actually be a massive overgrowth of yeast in the gut.

- Looking for any rise in candida antibodies in the blood, even within supposedly "normal" levels, still results in 10 percent false negatives. Another problem with a blood test is that it does not tell you what is happening now because antibodies may be present due to a previous yeast overgrowth.

- It is possible to test for candida based on whether you are a secretor or nonsecretor (your secretor status, explained below, is something you can establish using a home-test kit available from www.4yourtype.com/secretor-status -collection-kit/). We all have a blood type, either A, B,

AB, or O, and most people (about 75 to 80 percent) secrete minute amounts of chemical markers of their blood type into their normal secretions (such as saliva or mucus). The 20 to 25 percent or so of us who are non-secretors, irrespective of blood type, are known to have a greater tendency to have infections of all sorts, and yeast in particular. Women with recurrent vulvovaginal candidiasis, for example, are much more likely to be nonsecretors. Nonsecretors also process sugars less efficiently than secretors, adding to the likelihood of yeast overgrowth. People who have type O blood, particularly if they are nonsecretors, are far more likely to develop oral candidiasis.

- Gut fermentation tests are based on a blood sample taken before and after a sugar dose, on an empty stomach. The test assesses the quantity of ethanol or methanol produced in the next hour, giving an indication of yeast levels in the gut.

- Pain behind the sternum (breastbone) or thrush in the mouth are reliable signs of candida. However, breastbone pain is absent in 50 percent of people and thrush is not present in 30 percent of people who die of candidiasis. If these symptoms are present, together with other general signs of yeast overgrowth, then systemic candidiasis is strongly indicated.

- A low continuous fever for four days or more that fails to respond to antibiotic therapy is one of the signs of systemic candidiasis. In one study on septicemia in patients with leukemia, of the sixteen patients with this symptom who were treated for candidiasis, eleven became free of fever rapidly.

- The person's health history (such as antibiotic use) and the way apparent yeast-related symptoms respond to simple strategies such as markedly reducing sugar intake can be a pragmatic way of confirming candida activity. A self-assessment questionnaire, provided in chapter 4, provides a dependable guide as to whether or not candida is currently active. This suggests that the way to prove that a condition (or cluster of conditions) is the result of candida is to use a treatment that reduces yeast activity. If the symptoms then improve significantly or disappear altogether, the suggestion that yeast was at least part of the cause of symptoms would be difficult to contest.

- The Organix Dysbiosis test (made by Nordic Laboratories) is a urine organic acids test measuring the byproducts of microbial metabolism and is particularly useful in detecting the presence of pathogenic microbial overgrowth such as the waste products of the candida yeast, known as D-arabinitol. An elevated test result strongly suggests an overgrowth of candida. This test also helps to determine if the candida overgrowth is in your upper gut or small intestines.

- One quick method for testing for candida is a vaginal self-test. Vaginitis is now one of the most common reasons for physician visits, and approximately 30 percent of all cases are caused by infection by *Candida albicans*. An accurate, inexpensive, ten-minute self-test or vaginal candida test is available by means of a medically validated product called SavvyCheck. Many pharmacies sell this over the counter, and it is also available online. The great usefulness of this particular test is that you can check your progress in reducing candida over time.

THE IMPORTANCE
OF ONE'S HEALTH HISTORY

While these signs and assessment methods may be useful in a clinical or hospital setting, in private practice or in self-assessment of candidiasis it is generally agreed that the medical history and presenting symptoms of the person are an accurate guide as to whether or not candida is presently active. Quite simply, the way to prove that a condition (or a cluster of conditions) is the result of candida proliferation is to treat as if it is. The proof is in whether the symptoms disappear. Candidiasis is one of the very few instances where the treatment of a health problem is in fact the main means of diagnosing the problem. For this reason it is critically important to be aware of all of the symptoms of candida overgrowth.

A careful medical history that looks at previous and current medical treatments and drug usage, as well as at diet and stress factors, will give clear indications as to the likelihood, or otherwise, of candida being a possible culprit. It is these areas that we are going to explore in this book in order to formulate recommendations for the control of candida and for the prevention of its complications.

The potentially disastrous health damage caused by the exaggerated activity of an otherwise fairly harmless yeast that is normally easily tolerated and controlled is one of the complications of modern civilization. Candidiasis is fast becoming so widespread as to constitute an epidemic. The failure, thus far, by all but a handful of doctors to recognize this situation is tragic, for the degree of human suffering involved is enormous. Prevention is not difficult, and control, while a relatively slow process (taking months, not years), is not beyond the abilities of any intelligent person.

I earlier noted the pioneering work on candida by C. Orion Truss, particularly in his book *The Missing Diagnosis*. Another pioneer in this field is William Crook, a pediatrician and the author of thirteen books, including *The Yeast Connection* and *The Yeast Connection and Women's Health*. Both of these books suggest for their attack on yeast the use of an antifungal drug called nystatin, as well as other methods, including those involving nutrition and desensitization. This book, however, will not attempt to echo the drug approach suggested by these two practitioners, but instead it presents nondrug alternatives to the use of nystatin. This is not to say that nystatin and other antifungal drugs should never be used—only that in most cases there are other, safer ways of restoring the competence of the body to fight the yeast. There are many sound reasons for trying to find drug alternatives (as will be explained in later chapters), including many naturally occurring nutrients that enhance the control of the wildly proliferating yeast without producing resistant strains, something now thought likely when nystatin is used for long periods. This is the only reason I have taken this approach, for in every other way the two aforementioned books are excellent and valuable contributions to the growing body of literature on candida.

Let's next take a closer look at the nature of candida—what makes it active and how to recognize such activity. After that we will begin to learn how to deal with it.

LITERATURE

Crook, William. *The Yeast Connection*. New York: Vintage, 1986.

———, Carolyn Dean, and Elizabeth Crook. *The Yeast Connection and Women's Health*. New York: Square One, 2007.

Fotos, P. G., and J. W. Hellstein. "Candida and candidosis: Epidemiology, diagnosis and therapeutic management." *Dental Clinics of North America* 36, no. 4 (1992): 857–78.

Odds, Frank C. "Candida infections: An overview." *Critical Reviews in Microbiology* 15, no. 1 (1987): 1–5.

———, P. Auger, P. Krogh, A. N. Neely, and E. Segal. "Biotyping of *Candida albicans:* results of an international collaborative survey." *Journal of Clinical Microbiology* 27, no. 7 (1989): 1506–9.

Reizenstein, P. "Systemic candidiasis." *The Lancet* 329, no. 8527 (1987): 275.

———. "Systemic candidiasis in patients with hematologic diseases." *Scandinavian Journal of Infectious Diseases* 16 (1978): S44–S45.

———, M. Penchansky, B. Lantz, et al. "Prevention of septicemia and early death in acute leukaemia." *Current Chemotherapy* (1978): 248–50.

Ruhnke, M. "Epidemiology of *Candida albicans* infections and role of non–*Candida albicans* yeasts. *Current Drug Targets* 7, no. 4 (2006): 495–504.

Truss, C. Orion. *The Missing Diagnosis*. C. Orion Truss, 1983 (out of print).

———. *The Missing Diagnosis II*. C. Orion Truss, 2009.

CHAPTER 2

Candida and
Your Immune System

There is strong evidence to suggest that systemic fungal infections—those that affect the organs and tissues of the body—have increased dramatically in both frequency and severity in recent years. A recent multicenter survey identified *Candida* as the most common health care–associated bloodstream pathogen in the United States. For example, in the United States fungal infections of the bloodstream increased by over 200 percent between 1979 and 2000, while the number of deaths in the United States, in which yeast-related blood infections were listed on the death certificate, increased 400 percent between 1980 (1,557 deaths) and 1997.

The reasons for these dramatic increases in systemic fungal infections are attributed to advances in the treatment of serious diseases and the ongoing human immunodeficiency virus (HIV) epidemic, which have expanded the population of people with weakened host defenses against infections, as well as the widespread availability and overuse of antibiotics. It is therefore imperative that we understand how to help the body protect itself from yeast overgrowth.

THE BODY'S SELF-HEALING CAPABILITY

Whenever we are ill we experience the unpleasant symptoms of the illness. However, symptoms are often signs that the body is fighting the actual cause of the condition. For example, if you have an infection, your temperature goes up—a clear sign that your immune system is fighting the infection. It is important to learn to understand symptoms and not to fight them, but instead to deal with the underlying cause of the illness. Another example would be the multiple symptoms of digestive distress, which can include heartburn, bloating, constipation, and diarrhea. There are medications that relieve these symptoms, albeit temporarily, but such medications will not deal with the underlying cause of the digestive issue—and often these kinds of drugs only make matters worse in the long run.

There is one constant trend through sickness and health, and that is the body's self-healing, self-regulating, homeostatic tendency. Your many interacting body systems (including the immune system) constantly strive for homeostasis. Cuts heal, breaks mend, and infections are self-limiting (usually without any outside help). Diarrhea and vomiting, however unpleasant, are the means by which the body gets rid of toxic substances. Instead of trying to mask symptoms, we should learn to recognize and understand the body's self-regulation message in order to learn what causes symptoms. We also need to beware of the many things we do that can aggravate and strain the defense systems of the body, retarding healing and recovery.

Where infection is concerned, the ideal outcome is that the bacteria, virus, or yeast is contained and overwhelmed by the homeostatic defenses of the body. Unfortunately, when your self-repair mechanisms have to deal with too many demands at the same time, or when they are weakened, they may not always be able to achieve that outcome. The following factors should be considered:

- Are you getting enough essential nutrients in your diet?
- Are you eating a poor diet loaded with refined carbohydrates and sugars?
- Are you getting adequate exercise?
- Have you picked up a viral or yeast infection that never completely goes away?
- Are you not sleeping well?
- Are you experiencing work or emotional stress?
- Do you have a slight hormonal imbalance?
- Do you have a history of antibiotic use?
- Do you take contraceptive pills?

Each of these factors may be relatively minor, such that a person could cope with them or eliminate them by eating more sensibly, getting more exercise and sleep, doing something positive about job-related or emotional stress, or getting treatment for hormonal, viral, and yeast problems. But if nothing is done and these various adaptive demands (and others) continue, the body's defense and repair systems eventually become so overloaded that chronic symptoms are likely to appear. And, of course, whatever emotional stress, nutritional deficiencies and acquired toxicities, and biomechanical stresses (e.g., poor posture, tense muscles, poor breathing habits) there may be add to the overall stress load, which is managed within the context of the unique genetic characteristics of each person (such as secretor status, mentioned in chapter 1). It seems that some people have an inborn ability to handle their stress load more efficiently than others, so that their symptoms, and the severity of those symptoms, are not as pronounced or as long-lasting as they are in other people. So what is the solution?

Essentially there are three options:

1. Reduce adaptive demands. For example, stop and reverse the factors causing the demands that are overloading the body's ability to cope.
2. Focus on methods that help the repair and support systems of the body, to allow them to more efficiently handle the stress load.
3. Treat the symptoms—because sometimes this is all that's possible.

If the right changes are made, the body's innate homeostatic defense mechanism should be able to begin to work more efficiently once again, to detoxify, fight infection, and rebuild and repair, and at this point symptoms should gradually ease.

Some of the strategies needed to recover from a candida overgrowth could involve any or all of the following:

- Ensure optimal nutrition; remove toxins (however tasty) and increase nutritionally whole foods.
- Learn to handle stress more effectively.
- Take immediate action to deactivate yeasts or other organisms.
- Rebalance hormonal status and the chemistry of the body

through such agents as vitamins, minerals, trace elements, and amino acids.

- Detoxify the system, particularly the liver.
- Start to heal the lining of the intestines, which may have been damaged by an overgrowth of yeast.
- Do whatever else that may be needed to help reduce the adaptive demands that are overloading the homeostatic systems.

ABOUT CANDIDA

Candida albicans is a member of the class in the kingdom of fungi known as Saccharomycetes. Yeasts live practically everywhere on the planet and can derive their nutrients from most organic sources. This means that anything that is alive or has been alive can support yeasts. Rather than having roots like other plants, yeasts can derive their nutrients via the enzymes they produce. Given the right conditions for growth and replication, a yeast is capable of explosive growth, as anyone who has made bread will testify.

Candida is a yeast that lives inside everyone. It seldom takes over a person's entire body, but when it does the consequences are horrific. It can only achieve such a disproportionate state if the environment for its growth is excellent, and if the body's naturally regulating defense mechanisms are severely compromised or absent. It is important to realize that candida is an opportunistic fungus, not a pathogenic one. This means that it can live in your body without causing any problems whatsoever—unless and until an opportunity arises that allows it to become explosively active. This is more likely when your immune system is less efficient—when you are run down, stressed, poorly nourished, or when your internal control system, which consists mainly of the healthy bacteria in your gut, is depleted or damaged, such as what occurs following the use of antibiotics or steroids.

Not Only *albicans* Species

Candida albicans is the cause of most serious candida infections, but there are a number of other candida species that are becoming increasingly involved in yeast-related diseases. This happens mainly in people with compromised immune systems—for example, those taking immunosuppressive medication following transplants.

Research into the origin of candida bloodstream infections in the United States between 1998 and 2000 showed that *Candida albicans* was the cause of 45 percent of cases, followed by *Candida glabrata* (24 percent), *Candida parapsilosis* (13 percent), *Candida tropicalis* (12 percent), and other candida species (6 percent). Note that all of these species can live harmlessly in the intestinal tract or vagina, except *C. parapsilosis,* which lives on the skin.

Candida's Environment

Candida favors the digestive system, largely living in the intestines. It also likes to occupy sites in the vaginal region, in the mouth, and on the skin. It can live in all these places without causing any symptoms, as long as general health and immune function are good.

Research has shown that almost everyone has antibodies to candida. When such antibodies are present this indicates that the person's immune system has been challenged to respond to the presence of the yeast. In his book *The Missing*

Diagnosis, Dr. Truss states that by the age of six months, at the latest, candida lives in or on at least 90 percent of people, as evidenced by a positive skin-test reaction when extracts of candida are injected just under the skin. This reaction shows that there has been a previous presence of the yeast to which the body has developed defensive antibodies. The fact that candida is in all of us, and yet many people sail through life with no apparent ill effects, indicates that we have learned to cope with our uninvited yeast "passengers." Unlike certain other minute creatures that live in the digestive tract and serve a beneficial purpose, such as *Lactobacillus acidophilus* (which helps with the breakdown of food and helps in the synthesis of some of the B vitamins), there is no symbiotic relationship with candida. There is no trade-off, whereby a "room" in the "house" is given in exchange for something useful. So candida is, pure and simple, a parasite, a freeloader. This is perhaps inevitable in terms of the multitude of opportunistic microscopic creatures in both the animal and vegetable kingdoms. Most, if not all, plants and animals enjoy similar relationships with bacteria and fungi. Some of these relationships are mutually beneficial and some are distinctly one-sided. So candida, for all the musicality of its name, is an unwelcome boarder and a potential danger throughout life.

Once we know just what sort of situations remove our ability to control candida naturally, giving it the chance to proliferate by virtue of an environment conducive to its growth, we can begin to understand what needs to be done to contain it when it gets out of hand and starts producing health problems. And part of the solution involves coming to an understanding of the ways in which the body has learned to take care of the threat of parasites. It may be that we cannot actually stop candida from taking up squatter's rights in the body, but we can certainly confine its activities to a small and relatively safe part of the premises.

THE BODY'S
AMAZING DEFENSIVE CAPABILITY

Let's take a look at the body's amazing defensive capability. It has long been observed that people who survive certain infections seldom suffer from that same disease again. It's because they develop antibodies to the infecting organism. Apart from conferring such specific resistance to various disease-causing microorganisms, the immune system plays a vital role in other biological reactions.

In relation to fighting infection we have, in essence, two systems of defense. One is based on the thymus gland, which lies just below the breastbone and produces T cells. The other part of the immune system is made up of different types of white blood cells, called B cells. These protect you from most bacterial invaders and some viral infections. By producing antibodies, B cells neutralize many potential enemies. The two systems together make up the surveillance and protection agency of the body and work in harmony—with the thymus, it is thought, taking the leading role.

The white blood cells, which act as the soldiers in the front line of the battle, are manufactured mainly in the marrow of the long bones of the body. Some of these are actually turned into T cells by the influence of hormones from the thymus gland. Other white blood cells are turned into lymphocytes. Anything that tries to get into the bloodstream or into the interior of the body has to contend with the defensive

T and B cells and their powerful ability to neutralize foreign substances or organisms. If a B cell senses a foreign organism, it produces antibodies that are specific to the invader. At the same time, other B cells are alerted as to the alien presence, which causes them to manufacture antibodies to destroy the enemy.

It is believed that there are in excess of a million different kinds of antibodies in the bloodstream. As they are manufactured and deployed against the intruder, the lymphocytes go into action along with other white blood cells to dispose of the waste products of the battle between the intruder and the body. Thus a condition such as influenza is self-limiting, in that the fever and the symptoms of aching represent the intense activity that is going on in the body to deal with the invading virus, as well as the effects of the resulting toxicity of the metabolic-breakdown products of the battle.

When T cells come across an invading organism, whether it be a virus or a fungus such as candida (or even a mutant cancer cell), they produce what are known as *lymphokines,* which can kill microorganisms (or cancer cells). One such lymphokine that has received much attention in recent years is interferon. Lymphokines can also call up assistance from some powerful allies in this battle, called *macrophages,* which eliminate microorganisms and tumor cells by literally swallowing them whole. Sometimes the T cells act as "helper" cells to the B cells in their production of antibodies to fight the invader. They can also act as suppressor cells to stop a defensive process from getting out of hand when there may be a danger of B or T cells actually attacking friendly tissues in the body.

What If the Immune System Is Inefficient?

When for any one of a number of reasons (which we will consider in a later chapter) the immune system becomes weakened, we say the person is immunodeficient, that is, having a poor immune response. It is when these valiant soldiers, the T and B cells, along with the macrophages and their various assistants, are in a weakened state that the silent "squatters" in the body become free of the constraints that the defense system normally imposes and spread to areas beyond their normal territory. At that point a vast array of problems and symptoms can arise.

This system of defense, with its checks and balances, may become disrupted to such an extent that the condition now known simply as AIDS may occur. This particular disease is, of course, the result of HIV virus infection—and represents the extreme of immune deficiency—from which we can learn a great deal about immune function. AIDS stands for "acquired immune deficiency syndrome," and in this condition it is the T cells (from the thymus gland) that function inadequately. In fact, the ratio between the helper and suppressor cells alters so that there is an excess of suppressor cells, in contrast with the situation that exists in normal health. Much research in the treatment of immune-related conditions focuses on methods that can enhance the function of the thymus gland so that it can produce a balanced and adequate supply of active T cells. Among the nutrient factors that we can use to this end are vitamin C and the amino acid arginine. The amounts of these supplements used in treating conditions like AIDS, where the immune system is severely disrupted, are very large indeed (upward of 20 grams of vitamin C daily, and 3 to 5 grams of arginine). We'll be taking a detailed look at supplementation to benefit the immune system in a later chapter of this book.

How Candida Can Trick the Immune System

Autoimmune conditions occur when for various reasons the body's immune system attacks itself, for example, celiac disease, an inflammatory condition affecting the small intestine, as well as some skin diseases, such as dermatitis herpetiformis. This "error" may occur in people who are genetically sensitive to gluten (found in wheat and other grains) because of the similarity of the gluten protein to those that candida uses to attach itself to the gut lining, known as Hwp1, or Hyphal wall protein 1. This severe bowel disease can therefore be a real example of mistaken identity.

Systemic Infection

In recent years there has been an increase in incidences of widespread, systemic, candida-related infections, particularly in hospital settings, to wit:

- In Europe, in 2010, approximately 50 percent of systemic candida infections occurred in intensive-care units.
- In the United States, systemic fungal infections acquired during hospitalization increased by over 200 percent between 1980 and 2000.

At the same time, candida's resistance to the most widely used drugs (such as fluconazole) has increased. Thankfully, newer antifungal drugs (such as the echinocandins) are now available in cases of life-threatening infections. The general approach offered in this book, however, is to provide preventive as well as natural therapeutic recommendations. Quite simply, the more efficient your immune system is, the less likely it is that candida and other yeasts will be able to proliferate.

Can You "Catch" Candida?

You seldom "catch" or acquire yeast infections from an external source (although new strains can be introduced via sexual contact) because you have candida inside you (and possibly on your skin) for most of your life.

The most likely source of candida species in human disease is endogenous, that is, from inside of you, or from your own skin. Candidiasis arises in people who are predisposed because of illness, debility, or local reduction in resistance to overgrowth of their own yeast flora. The evidence gleaned from much research is that about half the healthy population (no illness or symptoms) have candida yeast in their mouths; this is easily assessed by means of a swab sample.

Levels of *Candida albicans* in the intestines of healthy people are described by researchers as high—between 30 and 60 percent. And in people who are ill, especially where immune function is weakened, levels of various *Candida* species are closer to 80 percent. Candida in the vagina is found in approximately 20 percent of healthy women and, when there is also vaginitis (inflamed tissues) present, the levels are much higher.

We can therefore see that when the immune system is in a weakened state, not only do yeast infections become more frequent, but the infecting agent may not need to be acquired from the outside, as it may quietly be biding its time in small amounts in your mouth, digestive tract, or vagina, waiting for your defenses to drop due to stress, infection, dietary indiscretions, or any of a host of other factors. If this happens, the ever-present, opportunistic yeast will seize the opportunity to slip through the defense barriers and advance to areas previously out of bounds.

This simplistic picture of what can happen contains the essential facts: Your body is self-healing. And if this self-healing ability, known as *homeostasis,* is weakened or overwhelmed, organisms such as yeasts, which are already inside you, can spread and wreak havoc.

The solution to this scenario is therefore twofold: (1) reduce the yeast (or other invading organism) activity; and (2) improve your defensive and self-healing potentials.

WHEN YEAST TAKES OVER

We know that before it becomes invasive the candida yeast alters to a different form, known as its *mycelial fungal form,* in which it has characteristics that make it more dangerous, such as a root structure that enables it to penetrate through mucosal barriers like those of the digestive tract, with a variety of harmful consequences resulting from the absorption of the products of digestion directly into the bloodstream.

Research by Dr. Truss indicates that many of the toxic effects of candida activity result from its ability to manufacture, under appropriate conditions, the substance known as *acetaldehyde* (produced by the partial oxidation of ethanol by the liver enzyme alcohol dehydrogenase). He points out that this well-known toxin could produce both the clinical and the laboratory characteristics of candida infection. To arrive at this conclusion, Dr. Truss analyzed the amino-acid profiles of affected persons. He maintains that this theory defines the symptoms of chronic yeast infection in terms of a toxin that common strains of candida can be shown to produce in laboratory conditions. This provides the chemical link between normal yeast fermentation and the metabolic abnormalities found in susceptible individuals. Dr. Truss stresses that it is highly probable that the symptoms experienced by many candida sufferers relate directly to the ability of yeast to ferment sugar into acetaldehyde in the body.

There are now tests that measure any rise in blood alcohol levels after a "sugar loading," in which alcohol (such as acetaldehyde) is measured after taking a specific amount of sugar on an empty stomach. This "gut fermentation" test is not foolproof, however, for a number of reasons, including the fact that other organisms, including certain bacteria that live in the gut, can also ferment sugar. Some laboratory technicians performing these tests (and many practitioners involved in treating chronic candidiasis) report being able to smell the alcohol on people who have eaten sugar and who never drink alcohol. In my own personal practice I have treated people for candidiasis who have been breathalyzed and found to be over the legal limit of alcohol in their bloodstream—despite their not having consumed any alcohol at all!

The Role of Amalgam Fillings in Immune-System Depression

There is substantial evidence that immune-system depression can result from mercury toxicity in the body via amalgam fillings in the teeth. Studies have shown there are several ways in which this highly toxic metal is able to enter the body, with resulting harmful effects on the immune system. And when the immune system is depleted it is vulnerable to the spread of candida. There are many dentists today who are willing to help affected patients by removing mercury amalgams and replacing them with either composite or gold fillings.

Although the relationship between amalgam fillings and health problems in general, and candida involvement in particular, is still incomplete, there is ample evidence that candidiasis is the most common fungal infection in the human mouth, with 85 percent of cases caused by *Candida albicans* adhering to amalgam and composite fillings, and that oral candidiasis is more common in people with amalgam fillings.

Replacing existing fillings may be required in cases where a strong link can be established between a health condition and measurable mercury toxicity resulting from dental amalgams. The use of supplemental amino-acid compounds such as glutathione, along with vitamin C, can help to ease mercury deposits out of the body. Tests can be done to measure your sensitivity to mercury, and also to measure the levels of mercury in your mouth (escaping in the form of a gas), as well as the electrical activity in the teeth that is set up by the combination of different metals used in amalgam fillings. These methods, as well as hair analysis, another way to measure the level of mercury, can all indicate just how significant a problem this could be.

The Importance of Dental Hygiene

A further dental hazard related to candidiasis was discovered in a study that looked at fifty patients with respiratory disease who had all developed candidiasis in the mouth and pharynx. Thirty-two of the subjects wore dentures, and this was thought to be a major factor in the onset of candida overgrowth (among the other factors were cortisone and antibiotic use, and the use of immunosuppressive sedatives). Researchers concluded that "dentures cause tissue trauma, provide sites for [yeast] colonization and diminish salivary flow. Saliva is necessary for normal oral immune defence." It was found that if dentures were treated with antifungal chemicals, this helped prevent this hazard. Regular sterilizing of dentures is suggested as a safe preventive measure, along with oral rinsing with diluted aloe vera juice.

A 2012 study looked at 140 subjects to determine the relationship between oral hygiene and colonization of *Candida* species in the oral cavity. Researchers concluded the following:

> Candida species were identified in 28.6% of respondents. The most present were *Candida albicans,* in 85% of cases. The presence of plaque, tartar and high index oral hygiene (IOH) in patients with *Candida* is statistically significant. It was found that 83.4% of patients with *Candida* poorly maintained oral hygiene. Poor oral hygiene is associated with a significantly higher score in the presence of tartar, plaque and high IOH. In total 67% had amalgam fillings. The presence of amalgam fillings in patients with identified Candida was statistically significant.

Other Factors that Encourage Candida

In chapter 3 we will examine in depth the reasons why candida gets out of hand. For now I will summarize some of the most common causes behind the spread of yeast. Sugar, as we know, plays a critical role; so does toxicity resulting from mercury (and other heavy metals). Other factors include:

Age: As we get older, immune function declines, and yeast takes advantage of this.

Serious illness: In cases of illnesses like diabetes, cancer/leukemia, asthma, and autoimmune diseases, the illness itself may be associated with a declining immune efficiency (cancer, for example), or the medication or treatment used may encourage yeast to spread (steroids used to treat asthma such as cortisone, or antibiotics).

Use of catheters after surgical procedures or trauma: This offers yeast an easy access to the bloodstream unless hygiene is scrupulous.

Radiotherapy: This severely lowers immune efficiency in the tissues affected.

Low levels of stomach acid (achlorhydria): This encourages both bacterial and yeast colonization of areas where the acid would normally prevent colonization.

Pregnancy: Hormonal changes might be involved in complex changes influencing immune function during pregnancy, particularly, as researchers Mor and Cardenas report in their 2010 study, "the pregnant woman's susceptibility to and severity of certain infectious diseases."

Use of the contraceptive pill or hormone-replacement therapy: These alter the ecology of parts of the body, allowing candida to spread.

Anything that reduces the efficiency of the intestinal flora ("friendly bacteria"): This includes prolonged stress and a diet high in fat and/or sugar and alcohol.

Our efforts to neutralize and control the spread and effects of candida (we can seldom get rid of it completely) depends on the use of whatever safe methods we have at our disposal to deprive it of its ideal nutrients, while at the same time building up and enhancing the depleted immune system. The immune system can then get on with the job of keeping candida in check. If we are to do more than temporarily suppress candida we must take this dual approach. The use of an antifungal drug will, it is true, in time destroy a great deal of candida's potency and reduce its symptoms. However, this recuperative process will stop the moment the drug is no longer taken.

ANTICANDIDA PROTOCOL

The solution to controlling candida in the long term lies in a multipronged strategy that simultaneously

- deprives the yeast of its optimum nutrient environment ("starves" the yeast);
- actively kills yeast using safe, nontoxic methods;
- actively focuses on restoring the body's normal controls over yeast by supporting the immune system and encouraging a healthy intestinal flora;
- helps to restore damaged tissues, such as the mucous membrane of the digestive tract.

As we shall see, there are other methods that can help as well, such as altering the ability of the yeast to multiply. We will consider all of these natural, safe alternatives to the use of drugs in chapters 5 and 6.

What about Antifungal Drugs?

It is beyond question that there are conditions in which the use of antifungal drugs is necessary, especially in the case of a severe, life-threatening situation, or when the process of recovery would involve a very long period of time. In the main, however, once we learn to recognize the symptoms that indicate that candida is getting out of hand, the natural, nondrug approach that I suggest here will work, and work quite well.

With this in mind, the following modern drugs are all used effectively against various candida infections, depending on where the infection is primarily located (for instance, urinary tract, vagina, skin, or systemic): fluconazole (Diflucan), itraconazole (Sporanox), ketoconazole (Nizoral), miconazole (Daktarin, Femeron), amphotericin B (Fungilin), and flucytosine (Alcobon). The side effects of these drugs are minimal, especially if only a single dose is prescribed (which is often the case with medications such as fluconazole). The more severe reactions listed below should be seen in context, as the medication would typically only be used in cases of severe systemic candidiasis, when the person is very ill.

When the use of antifungal drugs is prolonged or repeated, the chances of side effects increase.* These include:

- Nausea, headache, and stomach discomfort (fluconazole, itraconazole)

---

*Note that it is important to always read the details of indications, contraindications, and possible side effects on all medications, whether prescribed or over-the-counter.

- Liver dysfunction, severe allergies (ketoconazole, although rarely)
- Severe pruritus (itching), gastrointestinal symptoms, fever (miconazole, especially at high doses)
- Fever, headache, backache, vomiting, thrombophlebitis, and, in some cases, irreversible kidney damage (amphotericin B)
- Nausea, vomiting, diarrhea, and (rarely) fatal liver disease (flucytosine)

Nystatin was one of the main antifungals used before the availability of the modern drugs listed above. Nystatin, like amphotericin B, is derived from the fermentation of the fungus *Streptomyces albulus* or *S. noursei*. It is considered relatively safe and nontoxic, although Dr. Truss and others report that once it is stopped, when candida is apparently under control, a rebound of yeast activity can be anticipated unless a broad anticandida program has been adopted.

Nystatin is effective against certain candida strains while others are resistant. Not being a broad-spectrum antifungal agent, it allows for the proliferation of yeasts such as *Trichophyton* spp. (which cause athlete's foot, ringworm, jock itch, and similar infections of the nails, beard, skin, and scalp), which are resistant to it while the candida is attacked. This can lead to opportunistic overgrowth of these resistant yeasts even though the candida yeast is controlled in the short term.

The unfortunate aspect of most antifungal drug treatments is that they are seldom used together with a comprehensive antifungal dietary and supplement approach, which would encourage a healthier digestive tract and immune system in the long run.

Drugs are seldom necessary at all unless the infection is severe and widespread, since the methods I outline in later chapters are safer and of proven efficacy.

SUMMARY

- Let us not lose sight of the fact that candida lives in each and every one of us, and that it usually produces no symptoms unless the host environment has been compromised.
- Diagnosis of yeast involvement in health problems is not a case of establishing whether or not yeast is present—because it always is, to some extent. Rather, it is the task of the health care provider who is advising anyone with yeast-related problems to attempt to discover what underlying factors have allowed yeast to proliferate, and to focus attention on these, as well as to control fungal activity.
- Any approach that targets the yeast alone will result in a return of symptoms sooner rather than later. It is not just the yeast that we need to control, but the underlying causes that have allowed it to opportunistically explode into action.

We will now go on to consider just what can happen to weaken your wonderful defense mechanism, the immune system, as well as additional ways in which candida is sometimes allowed to go on a rampage, and so begin to colonize other areas of the body.

LITERATURE

Alangaden, George J. "Nosocomial fungal infections: Epidemiology, infection control, and prevention." *Infectious Disease Clinics of North America* 25, no. 1 (2011): 201–25.

Centers for Disease Control, U.S. "Invasive Candidiasis Statistics." www.cdc.gov/fungal/diseases/candidiasis/invasive/statistics.html.

Delaloye, Julie, and Thierry Calandra. "Invasive candidiasis as a cause of sepsis in the critically ill patient." *Virulence* 5, no. 1 (2014): 161–69.

Fidel, Paul L., Jr., Jose A. Vazquez, and Jack D. Sobel. "*Candida glabrata:* Review of epidemiology, pathogenesis, and clinical disease with comparison to *C. albicans*." *Clinical Microbiology Reviews* 12, no. 1 (1999): 80–96.

Geffers, Christine, and Petra Gastmeier. "Nosocomial infections and multidrug-resistant organisms in Germany: Epidemiological data from KISS (the Hospital Infection Surveillance System)." *Deutsches Ärzteblatt International* 108, no. 18 (2011): 320.

Giri, S., and A. J. Kindo. "A review of *Candida* species causing blood stream infection." *Indian Journal of Medical Microbiology* 30, no. 3 (2012): 270–78.

Hajjeh, R. A., A. N. Sofair, L. H. Harrison, G. M. Lyon, B. A. Arthington-Skaggs, S. A. Mirza, M. Phelan, et al. "Incidence of bloodstream infections due to *Candida* species and in vitro susceptibilities of isolates collected from 1998 to 2000 in a population-based active surveillance program." *Journal of Clinical Microbiology* 42, no. 4 (2004): 1519–27.

Marinoski, Jovan, Marija Bokor-Bratić, and Miloš Čanković. "Is denture stomatitis always related with candida infection? A case control study." *Medicinski glasnik* 11, no. 2 (2014): 379–84.

Martin, G. S., D. M. Mannino, S. Eaton, et al. "The epidemiology of sepsis in the United States from 1979 through 2000." *New England Journal of Medicine* 348, no. 16 (2003): 1546–55.

Mascellino, M. T., G. Raponi, A. Oliva, C. M. Mastroianni, and

V. Vullo. "Candidaemia in immune-compromised hosts: Incidence and drugs susceptibility." *Journal of Clinical and Experimental Pathology* 2, no. 6 (2012): 102–8.

McCarty, T. P., and P. G. Pappas. "Invasive Candidiasis." *Infectious Disease Clinics of North America* 30, no. 1 (2016): 103–24.

McNeil, M. M., S. L. Nash, R. A. Hajjeh, et al. "Trends in mortality due to invasive mycotic diseases in the United States, 1980–1997." *Clinical Infectious Diseases* 33 (2001): 641.

Mor, G., and I. Cardenas. "The Immune System in Pregnancy: A Unique Complexity." *American Journal of Reproductive Immunology* 63, no. 6 (2010): 425–33.

Moran, G., D. Coleman, and D. Sullivan. "An introduction to the medically important *Candida* species." In *Candida and Candidiasis,* 4th ed., edited by R. A. Calderone and C. J. Clancy, 11–25. Washington, DC: ASM Press, 2012.

Muzurovic, S., E. Babajic, T. Masic, R. Smajic, and A. Selmanagic. "The relationship between oral hygiene and oral colonisation with *Candida* species." *Medicinski Glasnik* 11, no. 2 (2014): 415–17.

Pfaller, M. A., and D. J. Diekema. "Epidemiology of invasive candidiasis: A persistent public health problem." *Clinical Microbiology Reviews* 20, no. 1 (2007): 133–63.

Silva, S., M. Megri, M. Henriques, R. Oliveira, D. W. Williams, and J. Azeredo. "*Candida glabrata, Candida parapsilosis* and *Candida tropicalis*: Biology, epidemiology, pathogenicity and antifungal resistance." *FEMS Microbiology Reviews* 36 (2011): 288–305.

Staab, J. F., and B. Wong. "Fungal Infections, Systemic." In *Reference Module in Biomedical Research*. Elsevier, 2014.

Stein, Jay H., ed. *Internal Medicine.* 5th ed. Philadelphia, Pa.: Mosby/Elsevier, 1998.

Thompson, P., H. J. Wingfield, R. F. Cosgrove, B. O. Hughes, and M. E. Turner-Warwick. "Assessment of oral candidiasis in patients with respiratory disease and efficacy of a new nystatin formulation." *British Medical Journal* 292, no. 6537 (1986): 1699–1700.

Torres-Rodríguez, Josep M. "Invasive fungal infections." *Medicina Clínica* 110, no. 11 (1998): 416–18.

Truss, C. Orion. "Metabolic abnormalities in patients with chronic candidiasis: The acetal-dehydeypothesis." *Journal of Orthomolecular Psychiatry* 13, no. 2 (1984): 66–93.

———. *The Missing Diagnosis.* C. Orion Truss, 1983 (out of print).

———. *The Missing Diagnosis II.* C. Orion Truss, 2009.

Vincent, J. L., E. Anaissie, H. Bruining, W. Demajo, M. el-Ebiary, J. Haber, Y. Hiramatsu, et al. "Epidemiology, diagnosis and treatment of systemic *Candida* infection in surgical patients under intensive care." *Intensive Care Medicine* 24, no. 3 (1998): 206–16.

Windham, Bernard. "Mercury exposure levels from amalgam dental fillings: Mechanisms by which mercury causes over 30 chronic health conditions; results of replacement of amalgam fillings, and occupational effects on dental staff." *Medical Archives* 66, no. 6 (2012): 415–17.

Wisplinghoff, H., T. Bischoff, S. M. Tallent, H. Seifert, R. P. Wenzel, and M. B. Edmond. "Nosocomial bloodstream infections in U.S. hospitals: Analysis of 24,179 cases from a prospective nationwide surveillance study." *Clinical Infectious Diseases* 39, no. 3 (2004): 309–17.

CHAPTER 3

How Candida
Can Run Amok

There are a number of predisposing factors that can allow candida to get wildly out of control. To a greater or lesser extent these same factors may be involved in the more subtle spread of this pernicious yeast, which is the case for the majority of people affected by the sort of symptoms outlined in chapter 1.

FACTORS
IN YEAST OVERGROWTH

Anyone affected by yeast overgrowth is likely able to identify a number of interacting causes. Seldom will only one factor be involved. Among the main causes:

An underlying inherited or acquired deficiency of the immune system: As mentioned in chapter 1, people who are nonsecretors of their blood type are much more likely to be carriers of candida and to have problems with persistent infections. Anyone who has type O blood who is a nonsecretor will be the most vulnerable, since candida finds it easier to colonize (attach to) O blood type cells. As noted in chapter 1, it has been shown that women who experience recurrent vulvovaginal candidiasis (i.e., thrush) are much more likely to be nonsecretors.

Steroids (hormones) and antibiotic residues from consuming nonorganic animal products: Antibiotics and hormones are given to conventionally raised animals to speed up their growth and control their susceptibility to disease. Anyone who regularly consumes factory-farmed beef, pork, veal, and poultry will absorb large amounts of antibiotic and hormone residues. Antibiotic residues are also found in dairy products and eggs unless they are guaranteed organic. Even low-level intake of these foods over many years can have a negative effect on one's ability to control the growth of candida.

Blood-sugar imbalances: Conditions like diabetes and hypoglycemia (low blood sugar) encourage candida to take over. Diabetes involves higher levels of sugar in the blood than are safe. Yet many nondiabetics have fluctuating blood-sugar levels for various reasons, including such habits as nicotine use, high caffeine consumption, high stress levels, or simply a dietary intake of refined sugars and carbohydrates. The anti-candida diet outlined in chapter 6 is suitable for diabetics as well as those whose blood-sugar levels are unstable for other reasons.

DIABETES QUESTIONNAIRE

If your answers to the following questions suggest a tendency toward diabetes, you should request a check-up with your health care provider:

1. Is there a history of diabetes in your family (particularly insulin-dependent diabetes)?

2. Are you over forty and overweight?
3. Have you become excessively thirsty for no obvious reason?
4. Do you urinate more frequently than in the past (with no actual bladder infection)?
5. Has your appetite increased without any change in your activity levels?
6. As well as the symptoms described in questions 3, 4, and 5, do you find yourself excessively tired for no obvious reason?

If you answered "yes" to either of the first two questions and to at least one of the other questions, a check-up is called for to rule out the possibility of early-onset diabetes.

HYPOGLYCEMIA QUESTIONNAIRE

If your answers to the following questions suggest a tendency toward hypoglycemia (low blood sugar), you should consider consulting a nutritionist or dietician.

1. Do you tend to wake up feeling tired and feel more energetic after breakfast?
2. If a meal is delayed or you skip a meal, would you expect to feel edgy, shaky, and/or faint?
3. Do you crave sugar-rich foods?
4. Do you regularly (more than once daily) use tea, coffee, chocolate, soft drinks, alcohol, or cigarettes?

A "yes" answer to any of these questions suggests the possibility of low blood sugar. More than one "yes" strongly suggests this to be the case.

A variety of strategies can be followed to help normalize low blood sugar, including supplementing daily with 200 micrograms (mcg) of chromium (glucose tolerance factor), eating a diet rich in proteins and complex (unrefined) carbohydrates, avoiding sugar-rich foods and the sort of stimulants listed in question 4, and following a "grazing" pattern of eating small amounts but more frequently. If candida is already a problem, such dietary changes will help, but you should also follow the anticandida protocols outlined in chapters 5, 6, and 7.

IMMUNE-SYSTEM CONSIDERATIONS

As we have seen in the previous chapter, part of the body's response to an intruder such as candida is to produce antibodies to meet a particular antigen (a foreign substance that stimulates a response on the part of the immune system). Candida has many antigens, and the efficiency with which the defensive operation is carried out against any particular one of these antigens can to some extent be inborn (that is, genetic). There is great variation in the degree of response by any one person to the different antigens. This can lead to a situation in which the immune system, unable to counteract and expel the candida invasion adequately, tolerates it in increasing amounts.

Biochemical Individuality

We are each biochemically unique. This means that there are wide variations in the particular requirements for any of the over forty nutrients that we require for survival and health. Many of these individual needs are determined before birth, and this has led to the genetotrophic theory of disease causation. Simply put, this theory says that because a person has unique inborn requirements that may greatly vary from what might be considered "average" or "normal," there is a good chance that one or another of these needs are not being met by the normal dietary intake. This leads at best to a lowered degree of function and at worst to a deficiency disease.

To a large extent this individual genetic factor also applies to our ability to handle the pathogens or microorganisms that can infect us. This is certainly the case in one's ability to handle candida efficiently, as we saw in the earlier discussion of our secretor status, which is determined by a genomic test. It seems that since infestation by yeast is almost universal, we are incapable of totally controlling its presence in our bodies. Some people will be more able than others to keep it under control and limit its spread. Thus some people are tolerant of the spread of a certain amount of yeast in their body.

The commonest areas for this proliferation of yeast to occur are the mouth, the throat, and the vaginal area. If this initially produces a degree of reaction indicating activity on the part of the immune system, then we would likely see the manifestation of the condition called *thrush*—a yeast infection (caused by *Candida albicans*) that is characterized by thick white, lacy patches on top of a red base on the tongue, palate, or elsewhere inside the mouth. This flares up periodically when there may also be other factors involved that lower the body's general vitality. Eventually, in many cases, the condition might no longer evoke an acute flare-up but would remain in a semipermanent, chronic state. This happens when the body surrenders to the yeast's foothold and is no longer able to mount attacks on it. This is an indication of impaired or deficient immune function. Among the many aspects of our environment that can influence this are stress, nutritional inadequacy, and pollution, as well as the use of specific drugs that weaken the immune system further.

Drugs and Immune Function

Nowadays we are all familiar with the concept of tissue and organ transplantation as well as joint replacement, which involve the use of powerful drugs designed to prevent the body from rejecting the new foreign tissue or organ. These immunosuppressive drugs have a primary task of stopping the natural defenses from working as they naturally would—in other words, these drugs are designed to suppress the immune system. As a result, the risk of infection by disease organisms obviously increases. Drugs such as steroids (hormones) also have this effect. These are conventionally used for a variety of conditions, ranging from rheumatic disorders to asthma and hormonal imbalances. The most common use of steroids, however, is not in the treatment of disease but in the contraceptive pill. This common medication increases the ability of candida to proliferate, as we shall see later in this chapter.

Immune System Nutrient Support

There are a variety of nutrients that can assist in the normal functioning of the immune system, including certain vitamins and minerals that have antioxidant properties. This means that they are able to slow down or stop a process in which free radicals cause tissue damage. Free radicals are especially reactive molecules that have one or more unpaired electrons. These can be produced in the body by natural biological processes or introduced from the outside (as in tobacco smoke, toxins, or pollutants). Free radicals can damage cells, proteins, and DNA by altering their chemical structure. Particularly valuable antioxidant nutrients include vitamin C and vitamin E (together with selenium), as well as certain amino acids such as methionine, cysteine, and glutathione. Vitamin B_6 (pyridoxine), zinc, manganese, and other nutrients are also useful for immune-system maintenance. A detailed discussion of nutrients is found in chapter 5.

Stress and Immunity

Stress, which involves a repeated or constant state of anxiety and all that it entails in terms of depletion of vital nutrient reserves, along with imbalances of internal secretions and functions, is a major cause of immune incompetence.

A new interdisciplinary science, psychoneuroimmunology (PNI), studies the direct connection between our emotions and how efficiently—or otherwise—our immune system behaves. The evidence is that there is a very clear link between the mind and the body, and it operates through the body's defense system, which is meant to protect both. One of the ways in which this is most dramatically demonstrated is during periods of stress, when people become far more prone to infection. This indicates the lowered efficiency of the immune system at such times, along with the body's increased need for vital nutrients such as zinc and vitamin C.

The interaction between anxiety and stress, and nutritional imbalances, leads to the immune system being deprived of the ability to operate efficiently. If at the same time there is increased demand on the effective functioning of the immune system to meet the challenges of environmental or nutritional toxicity (pollution of air, cigarette smoke, alcohol, caffeine-rich drinks such as coffee, chocolate, and tea, etc.), then a complex picture emerges in which excessive demands, inadequate nutrition (with associated deficiencies), and perhaps drug usage (such as the contraceptive pill) all interact to weaken immune function. Stress management, therefore, becomes a primary goal when trying to encourage improved immunity.

WOMEN AND CANDIDA

Most people with candida problems are women, and most are under the age of fifty. Why is this so?

Imagine a modern young woman who has grown up in an era characterized by the common and widespread use of drugs like antibiotics and steroids. More than likely she has had antibiotics prescribed to her over the years for minor problems such as tonsillitis and ear infections. She may have then developed bladder infections (cystitis) from time to time and had a broad-spectrum antibiotic prescribed for this problem. She may have had acne as a teenager, most probably treated with antibiotics. Should she have had cause, she may have had steroids for asthma or some other condition. Going on the pill, and subsequently coming off it and becoming pregnant, might have further enhanced the chances of yeast spreading and would have caused more problems, such as the recurrence of acne and cystitis. It's worth noting that because of the hormonal changes that take place during pregnancy, a degree of control over candida is lost. Yeast, therefore, finds this a good time to expand its activities in the mother's body, while the unborn child could be exposed to a variety of antigens from the increased candida activity.

Missing from this picture are all the other variables: nutritional imbalances, which are common in modern society; pollution; excessive use of sugar-rich foods (which yeast loves); and stress factors in general. The picture emerges of a woman who is doing just about all that is humanly possible to bring about the ideal conditions for yeast to thrive.

Risk Factors for Women

Dr. Truss, who as we know did so much to bring the candida problem to light, was scathing in his condemnation of certain drugs that compound the candida problem for women. In *The Missing Diagnosis* he notes that antibiotics are often used unadvisedly, in cases in which they have no role to play at all. In this way incorrectly diagnosed viral and fungal conditions may be uselessly "treated" with antibiotics. This actually increases the likelihood of the condition worsening. The widespread use of tetracycline to treat acne is another major factor in the spread of candida. Dr. Truss insists that there is no way anyone suffering from candida problems can control that condition if she (or he) continues with tetracycline. In fact, in many cases acne is actually the direct result of candida infection, and it will only worsen rather than improve on such a treatment.

Dr. Truss also strongly advised against using the contraceptive pill. He points out that chronic vaginitis tends to be at its worst when progesterone levels are high, as in pregnancy, and the luteal (post-ovulation) phase of the menstrual cycle. As the hormone progesterone is an active component of the pill, it is likely responsible for the fact that fully 35 percent of women using the pill have acute vaginal candidiasis. Is Dr. Truss correct in this assessment? Various scientific investigations have confirmed his view that the pill, as well as intrauterine contraceptive devices, certain spermicides and condoms, and some habits of hygiene, clothing, and sexual practices (in addition to pregnancy, hormone replacement therapy, uncontrolled diabetes, immunosuppression, antibiotics, glucocorticoids use, and genetic predisposition) dramatically increase the risk of vaginal candida infection.

In a recent European study, cultures were taken from 576 women in a hospital outpatient setting to assess the influence of pregnancy, diabetes, contraceptive medication, and antibiotic use on yeast infections. The researchers reached the following conclusions: *Candida albicans* was the commonest yeast isolated, and it was most common in premenopausal women. Single women were more likely to have a candida infection than married women. Pregnancy caused a significant increase in the rate of candida infection compared to other yeasts. Women with diabetes experienced a far higher rate of yeast infection compared to nondiabetic women. Yeast infections of all sorts were quite common in oral-contraceptive users. And a woman's use of an antibiotic led to a significant increase in her subsequently developing a yeast infection, compared to women who did not use antibiotics.

In the same study, the 576 women with vaginal candidiasis who were observed exhibited the following symptoms:

- 495 (85.9 percent) had severe itching (pruritus);
- 381 (66.1 percent) had vaginal discharge;
- 179 (31.1 percent) experienced soreness;
- 29 (5.0 percent) women reported painful intercourse (dyspareunia).

FOOD AND CANDIDA:
EXCLUSION TESTING

Yeast thrives on carbohydrate-rich foods. This means that to control candida we must attempt to deprive it of its sustenance by limiting or eliminating altogether all sugar-rich foods and refined carbohydrates—if not permanently, at least for the duration of the anticandida diet. (The specific details of this will be outlined in the nutritional program that appears in chapter 6.) Regarding other foods—particularly those containing yeasts to which you may have become sensitive—a simple self-testing method can be helpful. This involves an exclusionary period of ten to fourteen days, during which all yeast-based foods are eliminated. During this time it is important to keep a careful symptom score, as provided in chapter 7. After this period of yeast-food elimination (it takes at least five days for all traces of the excluded food to be cleared by the body) you can introduce a "challenge," in which you eat a small amount of a yeast-based food (or a fragment of a yeast tablet) twice in one day, observing either or both of the following reactions: (1) Did your symptoms improve when not eating such foods? And (2) did your symptoms return when you reintroduced these foods? A "yes" answer to either question suggests that you should investigate further, and that you would probably benefit from leaving such foods out of your diet for a while.

The dietary items that are suspect if yeast is not well tolerated include the following yeast-containing foods: vinegar, alcoholic beverages, yeast extracts and spreads, mushrooms, and anything with a mold on it, such as certain cheeses like blue cheese. A comprehensive list of yeast-type foods can be found in chapter 6.

It should be clearly understood that avoiding particular foods is necessary only if you have become sensitized—and are therefore allergic or sensitive to—fungus-related substances. If not, there is no reason to add yet another restriction to an already complex program.

Once candida is brought under control, unless a yeast sensitivity or allergy exists there is no reason to keep to a strict prohibition on these foods, although the return of classic symptoms of candida activity (such as abdominal bloating or sudden extreme fatigue after eating one of the offending foods) will tell you if it is time to return to your avoidance strategy.

Just as foods that contain molds or fungi are considered undesirable, it may be found as well that symptoms are worse in humid, damp environments, in which mold and fungus spores are present in the atmosphere. Thus it is very important to eliminate from the home any areas of dampness, such as on walls, floors, etc.

An Anticandida Program Is Not Forever!

Candida gets out of hand because we allow it to. We may do so in ignorance, but it is folly to blame the yeast when we have the power to control it, as millions of people have come to realize. Once you begin to suspect that your many and varied symptoms may be the result of candida activity, it is time to grasp the problem firmly and take responsibility for the situation.

Candida will not go away on its own. Its current activity may be the result of any combination of factors that have allowed it to escape from the body's normal efficient control mechanisms. To get it back to where it belongs (or at least to where it can do the least harm), you need to restore your defense capacity to its optimum and stop doing all those things that are helping yeast to thrive. It's as simple as that. You can do this by your own efforts—by reforming your dietary habits, by using particular nutrient substances, and by reducing the overall levels of stress and pollution in your immediate environment. Once you have put candida in its place, you can relax your vigilance to a great extent, in the sense of allowing your diet to contain certain of the "undesirable" substances from time to time. But you should constantly be aware of the factors that allowed candida to advance in the first place and avoid these as stringently as possible.

The next chapter looks at the sorts of problems that candida can cause when it gets out of control. Be prepared for some surprises.

LITERATURE

Gonçalves, B., C. Ferreira, C. T. Alves, M. Henriques, J. Azeredo, and S. Silva. "Vulvovaginal candidiasis: Epidemiology, microbiology and risk factors." *Critical Reviews in Microbiology,* Dec. 21, 2015: 1–23.

Grigoriou, O., S. Baka, E. Makrakis, D. Hassiakos, G. Kapparos, and E. Kouskouni. "Prevalence of clinical vaginal candidiasis in a university hospital and possible risk factors." *European Journal of Obstetrics, Gynecology, and Reproductive Biology* 126, no. 1 (2006): 121–25.

Truss, C. Orion. *The Missing Diagnosis II.* C. Orion Truss, 2009.

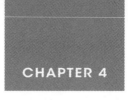

CHAPTER 4

Candida and Its Consequences for Your Health

The list of conditions in which candida is implicated as a major causative factor is very long indeed. There are literally dozens of health problems that are yeast-related, some minor (such as dandruff), but many that are disabling in their severity. How common are the commonest of such problems?

- Oral candida overgrowth (oropharyngeal colonization) is found in between 30 percent and 55 percent of healthy young adults.
- About 75 percent of American women experience vulvovaginal candidiasis at least once, and about 40 to 50 percent will experience more than one episode.
- The presence of *C. albicans* is detected in about 40 to 65 percent of normal fecal samples.

It is often necessary to deduce the involvement of candida from the history of the patient. (Have antibiotics been used? Is, or was, the contraceptive pill in use? Have cortisone or other steroids such as prednisone been prescribed?) The range and types of symptoms also give indications of candida's involvement. This is because it is virtually useless asking a microbiology lab to look for the presence of candida; we already know that it is present—to some degree—in practically all adults, and in most children within the first few months of life. Since we can usually conclude from the history and the symptoms when candida is likely to be the cause, what would a lab analysis prove? The proof of candida's involvement is obtained by carrying out an anticandida program and finding out whether or not this gets rid of most of the symptoms.

Michael T. Murray N.D. and Joseph E. Pizzorno N.D., authors of the *Encyclopedia of Natural Medicine,* say that the best way to diagnose candida-related problems is by means of clinical evaluation, combined with knowledge of yeast-related illness, a detailed medical history, and a patient questionnaire. In addition, there should be further tests to support the findings established by clinical evaluation.

CONDITIONS ASSOCIATED WITH CANDIDA

Before considering the major candida-related symptoms, let's look at the sort of conditions that are now known to be the possible result of candida's activity:

- Vaginitis (which may involve severe itching, burning, soreness, irritation, and discharge)
- Thrush (oral or vaginal, involving white patches on the mucosa)
- Endometriosis (a disorder involving the lining of the uterus)
- Athlete's foot

- Acne
- Dandruff
- Headache (migraine type)
- Fatigue
- Constipation
- Bloating
- Allergies
- Sensitivity to perfumes, fumes, chemical odors, and tobacco smoke
- Poor memory, feelings of unreality, irritability, inability to concentrate
- Depression
- Numbness, tingling, and weak muscles
- Painful muscles
- Heartburn
- Abdominal pain
- Diarrhea
- Irritable bowel syndrome
- Premenstrual syndrome
- Recurrent sore throats and nasal congestion
- Recurrent ear infections
- Swelling and discomfort in joints
- Blurred vision

Note: Almost all the conditions listed may be caused by factors other than candida, but all *might* involve yeast infection as a cause or aggravating feature—so how can you tell if yeast is the culprit?

The diagnosis of candida's involvement in any of these conditions becomes clearer if symptoms are aggravated during damp weather (or in damp places) or when in an environment with mold or fungus present. If the symptoms are worse after eating sugar-rich or fungus-containing foods, the evidence for candida's involvement becomes stronger yet.

LOCAL CANDIDA SYMPTOMS
START BEFORE GENERAL ONES

After we have looked at some of these conditions more closely, we will pull the key information together in the form of a questionnaire, which should enable you to assess the chances of candida being involved in your health make-up. In his article "Restoration of Immunological Competence to *Candida albicans*," Dr. Truss depicts the typical case of chronic candida infection. After pointing to the influence of multiple pregnancies, birth-control pills, antibiotics, and cortisone, as well as other factors that depress the immune system, he says:

> The onset of local symptoms of yeast infection, in relation to the use of these drugs, is especially significant and usually precedes the systemic response. Repeated courses of antibiotics and birth-control pills, often punctuated with multiple pregnancies, lead to ever increasing symptoms of mucosal infections in the vagina and gastro-intestinal tract. Accompanying these are manifestations of tissue injury, based on immunological and possibly toxic responses to yeast products released into the systemic circulation. Many infections are secondary to allergic responses of the mucous membranes of the respiratory tract, urethra and bladder, necessitating increasingly frequent antibiotic therapy that simultaneously aggravates, and perpetuates, the underlying cause of the allergic membrane that allowed the infection.

Depression is common, often associated with difficulty in memory, reasoning and concentration. These symptoms are especially severe in women, who in addition have great difficulty with the explosive irritability, crying and loss of self-confidence that are so characteristic of abnormal function of the ovarian hormones.

WOMEN, CANDIDA'S MAIN TARGET

Dr. Truss further points out that accompanying this sad catalog of ills are what he calls "poor end-organ response" resulting in acne, loss of libido (disinterest in sex), excessive menstrual bleeding and cramps, intolerance to foods and chemicals, and other problems. The typical (but by no means only) person suffering from candida infection is seen to be a woman somewhere between puberty and menopause who has undergone some, or all, of the predisposing factors (described in chapter 3) and who has some, or all, of the symptoms outlined in the quote above, a mixture of unaccountable vaginal and bowel symptoms, ranging from discharge and itching to bloating, discomfort, diarrhea, and/or constipation, as well as the emergence of an array of mental-emotional symptoms. In less enlightened times women suffering from such ills were labeled neurotic, and this is probably the crowning insult to the woman who has literally begun to feel her body and mind giving way in all directions.

DIGESTIVE TRACT COLONIZATION

The vaginal area and intestinal tract are commonly inhabited by candida, since they provide the damp atmosphere, and the nutrients, the fungus thrives on. If circumstances allow, candida can spread along the entire length of the digestive tract, from the anus to the mouth. The tongue may be coated, and there may be yeast deposits on the insides of the cheeks, the corners of the mouth, and the gums. White spots and a coating on the tongue are the obvious signs, accompanied by soreness and tingling of the gums. When the esophagus is affected it can result in symptoms commonly described as "heartburn," while indigestion and acid stomach are symptoms of candida's activity in the stomach. If the infestation is prolific in the small or large intestine, diarrhea can result, and it may be chronic and accompanied by mucus and/or blood. There may be cramplike and colicky pains—"spastic colon"—often associated with difficulty in having a normal bowel movement. Bloating and distension of the abdomen is a frequent occurrence with candida, and there may be a variety of abdominal noises as a result. If constipation is a factor, then hemorrhoids are a likely consequence, as is the possibility of rectal discomfort and itching.

WHAT HAPPENS WHEN
CANDIDA BECOMES A FUNGUS?

Candida is a dimorphic organism, which means that it has two quite separate identities, and that the very nature of candida changes under certain conditions. It can turn into its mycelial fungal form from its simple yeast form. In the simple yeast form it has no root, but in its fungal form it produces rhizoids, which are long structures similar to roots. The complication is that these "roots" can actually penetrate through the mucosa (lining) of the tissue in which they are growing.

One of the key controls that prevents this change is the abundant presence of the B vitamin biotin. In good health, biotin is manufactured in the intestines by friendly bacteria (known as probiotic organisms). After a person takes antibiotics (or anything else that upsets the function of *Lactobacillus acidophilus* or *Bifidobacterium bifidum*) these friendly bacteria may become severely depleted and unable to manufacture biotin. If this happens, control is removed from the yeast, and the aggressive fungal form emerges to start its onslaught on new territories in the body.

Supplementation with biotin helps to control this, as does restoration of normal bowel flora ecology via consumption of potent, viable strains of these friendly bacteria in the form of probiotic supplements. These are important and usually successful strategies in the campaign against candida. Until this control occurs, however, the change from yeast to fungus allows the fungal roots to breach the boundary between the body proper and the self-contained world of the digestive tract. This allows substances to enter the bloodstream that would otherwise have been kept out by this boundary. The fungal form of the candida organism is invasive, and it can use this avenue to enter the body proper.

Permeability

It would be a mistake to think that it is enough to simply swallow doses of friendly bacteria, in the form of probiotics, in the hope that this alone will rebalance the situation. Once damage has occurred to the mucous membranes of the intestines, the normal flora (such as *L. acidophilus* and *B. bifidum*) will have great difficulty in attaching to the intestinal lining, which requires a period of healing after the elimination of yeast, along with special strategies to help with this healing. (These strategies are detailed later in this book.)

The main problem that occurs when the intestinal barrier is broken by fungus is that undigested proteins from food eaten, as well as toxic wastes from the candida infestation, may begin to circulate in the bloodstream. And this is frequently the cause of a wide variety of symptoms, often of an allergic type.

Brain Allergies

If these metabolic waste products resulting from candida infection reach the brain, there is a chance that this will lead to what doctors Michael Murray and Joseph Pizzorno, authorities in natural medicine, call "brain allergies." These manifest in a wide variety of mood and personality problems ranging from depression, irritability, and mood swings, to conditions that look for all the world like the symptoms of schizophrenia.

Substances that enter the brain and act on the opiate receptors there to disrupt brain function and produce mental and personality symptoms are termed *exorphins*. They differ from endorphins, which are substances produced in the body that play a role in the functioning of many aspects of the biochemistry of life, including pain control. The externally originating substances (proteins from incompletely digested food, for example) that slip into the bloodstream through the gates opened by the fungal roots of candida can wreak havoc with whatever tissues they contact. They are seen as foreign invaders by the immune system, which will attempt to neutralize them. If such a process continues over a long period of time—and this sort of thing can go on for many years—then this in itself will contribute to the ultimate depletion of the immune function of the body. It simply becomes overwhelmed by the constant onslaught. The defensive reaction by the immune system to such substances may result in a wide range of what are seen as allergic reactions, including asthmatic attacks, nasal and respiratory conditions, skin reactions, palpitations, muscle and joint aches, swelling, and other symptoms.

Reproductive Organ Dysfunction

As noted earlier, the female reproductive organs are a major site for candida activity. If candida irritates the urethra it can be a cause of cystitis. If for any of a number of reasons the acidity of the region alters, then the relatively benign yeast form can alter into the fungal form and become active, spreading to other regions accessible from the vagina. This can lead to inflammatory conditions in the womb, fallopian tubes, and the ovaries themselves, the consequences of which can include infertility or sterility. Other symptoms can range from frequency of urination, coupled with a burning sensation, to chronic discharge, as well as premenstrual and menstrual problems, and the whole gamut of inflammatory and infectious involvements of the reproductive system.

What about PMS?

Premenstrual syndrome (PMS) is a set of emotional and physical symptoms that commonly start a week to ten days before menstruation. The symptoms usually stop when menstruation begins, or soon after.

Austrian researchers have found that use of anticandida medication (sertraline HCl) significantly reduces the symptoms of premenstrual syndrome (PMS). This seems to confirm what has long been suspected—that many of the symptoms of PMS are yeast-related.

Candida, the Mind, and the Emotions

The presence of mild to severe emotional and mental symptoms along with certain symptoms of ill health should alert you to the strong possibility of candida's activity. Often these mental/emotional symptoms are no more than a general feeling of being unable to concentrate, accompanied by memory lapses and feelings of lethargy and exhaustion. The symptoms may also be far more dramatic.

Dr. Truss says that many conditions are given names or labels simply because they fit into a pattern that is more or less recognizable as being similar to a particular known illness—as if a combination of symptoms that may have no obvious cause is somehow more medically manageable if it is labeled. In his book *The Missing Diagnosis* he reports on two patients who had been repeatedly diagnosed as schizophrenic, and another patient who was diagnosed as having multiple sclerosis. Dr. Truss points out that they all recovered on an anticandida treatment, and seventeen years later they were still in good health.

He asks, "Were two of these women really schizophrenic, or was it just that *Candida albicans* was responsible for brain function so abnormal that highly competent specialists never doubted the diagnosis of schizophrenia?" He further adds, "In the third woman, did *Candida albicans* induce neurological abnormalities sufficiently typical of multiple sclerosis that a competent neurologist would mistakenly diagnose the disease?" He answers these questions by saying that either the treatment dealt with a yeast infection, which can produce symptoms that mimic these diseases (and many others), or yeast can actually cause the diseases that are labeled as schizophrenia and multiple sclerosis. The indication, after many years of work by Dr. Truss and others, is that this is not just a case of remission (which is not uncommon in either schizophrenia or multiple sclerosis), but that candida induces symptoms similar to those of other illnesses, which may then be wrongly diagnosed and incorrectly labeled.

More recent research confirms the early work of Dr. Truss, showing that candida invasion of the central nervous system occurs in up to 50 percent of people with systemic candida (and other fungal) infections.

Candida and Chronic Fatigue Syndrome

Most people with chronic fatigue syndrome (also known as myalgic encephalomyelitis, or ME, and postviral fatigue syndrome) are infected with yeast overgrowth, and in many instances this is a major cause of their condition. It was learning about how the first edition of this book had changed someone's life that first drew my attention to this fact.

In 1986, Sue Finlay wrote in the London *Observer* about her symptoms—exhaustion, extreme muscle weakness, joint pain, mood disturbances, deteriorating eyesight, vague stomach problems—and related her long and frustrating search for a diagnosis. Finlay followed the anticandida regimen I recommended in the first edition of this book and credited it with making all the difference in her recovery from chronic fatigue syndrome. She tells of how her doctor, at her insistence, had already prescribed nystatin, and that this had taken her from "being confined to bed, hardly able to stand, tears all day and suicidal" to a point where "the feeling of being poisoned left me, a little energy returned." She then says that after some months of variable but gradual improvement,

> I came on the book *Candida Albicans: Could Yeast Be Your Problem?* by Leon Chaitow. I changed my diet radically. I cut out sugars and refined carbohydrates. All bread, mushrooms, tea, alcohol, vinegar, coffee, chocolate were dropped. All these foods feed the yeast. I used vitamin supplements to enhance my immune system, olive oil and garlic to attack the yeast and acidophilus powder to replace the Candida with healthy intestinal flora. I ate vegetables, salads, whole cereals and fruit in abundance. At present I am able to walk nearly half a mile without total collapse, I am beginning to work in the garden a little, I still have to rest every day and be careful not to overdo things and cause a relapse, but I have had eight months of improvement and am steadily reducing the nystatin.

It should be noted that only one thing needs correcting in Sue's account. Stopping yeast-based foods is not because they "feed" the candida yeast, but rather because the person will usually have become sensitized to yeasts as a result of *Candida albicans* infection, and therefore eating foods based on yeast or containing molds will further irritate and aggravate this situation.

Sue Finlay's condition continued to improve, and her message is the one I want people with chronic fatigue syndrome to take to heart. Your condition is *not* all in the mind. Chronic fatigue syndrome is more likely to cause depression than to be caused by it, and it is often largely the result of problems associated with an immune system that has been weakened by *Candida albicans* overgrowth.

UNDERSTANDING CANDIDA

It is clear that the ramifications of candida infection are not yet fully understood, and that much clarification and research remains to be done. In the meantime, since it is not difficult to identify reasons to suspect its possible involvement, it seems reasonable that a candida control program should be adopted regardless of whatever previous diagnosis has been made, in cases where a combination of both a history and symptoms of candida exist, and where there is a pattern of ill health similar to any of those touched on in this book. The treatment is, after all, not only harmless but in fact beneficial to one's overall health.

It's Not All in the Mind

Conditions that are linked to candida are frequently labeled "psychosomatic" illnesses. This can be a way for doctors to avoid having to say that they cannot find the cause. Calling patients' conditions "psychosomatic" may, if this diagnosis is repeatedly made, result in their beginning to believe that they really are not quite balanced. Terms like *neurotic* are often ascribed to someone who is suffering from the effects of widespread candida infection, and this can have devastating effects on morale and self-esteem. The yeast or fungal cause may remain totally unsuspected, or, if, for example, thrush is considered a part of the psychosomatic symptom picture, it may be simply regarded as a minor piece of the puzzle, unworthy of therapeutic focus.

Suggesting, as some have, that chronic fatigue syndrome is all in the mind angers many people afflicted by this condition and has led to patient self-help efforts and the demand for a more scientific consideration of this debilitating condition. Organizations such as Action for ME, which has done much in the United Kingdom for ME and chronic fatigue syndrome to be taken seriously, were in fact the result of frustration experienced by people like Sue Finlay, who hit a brick wall with the medical profession when told her problem was psychological. In the United States the National CFIDS Foundation (www.ncf-net.org) and the Solve ME/CFS Initiative (solvecfs.org) have grown out of the same frustration.

The questionnaire that follows will give you the chance to assess the possibility of candida being a major part of your current health picture. Note that it is possible for most of the symptoms described to be the result of causes other than candida. If, however, you have more than one of the indications on list 2, as well as some of the lesser symptoms found at the end of the questionnaire, then the possibility increases to a probability, especially if you can identify a possible causative link with at least one of the factors in list 1.

CANDIDA CHECKLIST

Completing the following questionnaire by responding to each question with either a "yes" or "no" answer will give you clues as to whether or not candida should be considered an active agent in your current health spectrum. It is not possible to make a diagnosis by these means alone, but a strong indication, as evidenced by positive answers in all sections of the questionnaire, can be used to assist you in deciding whether to undertake an anticandida regimen.

LIST 1: HISTORY OF DRUG USE

1. Have you ever taken a course of antibiotics for an infectious condition for eight weeks or longer, or for shorter periods four or more times in one year?
2. Have you ever taken a course of antibiotics for the treatment of acne continuously for a month or more?
3. Have you ever had a course of steroid treatment such as prednisone, cortisone, or ACTH?
4. Have you ever taken the pill (contraceptive medication) for a year or more?
5. Have you ever been treated with immunosuppressant drugs?
6. Have you been pregnant more than once?
TOTAL "Yes":

LIST 2: MAJOR SYMPTOM HISTORY

1. Have you in the past had recurrent or persistent cystitis, vaginitis, or prostatitis?
2. Have you a history of endometriosis?
3. Have you had thrush (oral or vaginal) more than once?
4. Have you ever had athlete's foot or a fungal infection of the nails or skin?
5. Are you severely affected by exposure to chemical fumes, perfumes, tobacco smoke, etc.?
6. Are your symptoms worse after taking yeasty or sugary foods or drinks?
7. Do you suffer from a variety of allergies?

8. Do you commonly suffer from abdominal distension, bloating, diarrhea, or constipation?
9. Do you suffer from premenstrual syndrome (fluid retention, irritability, etc.)?
10. Do you suffer from depression, fatigue, lethargy, poor memory, or feelings of unreality?
11. Do you crave sweet foods, bread, or alcohol?
12. Do you suffer from unaccountable muscle aches, tingling, numbness, or burning?
13. Do you suffer from unaccountable aches and swelling in joints?
14. Do you have vaginal discharge or irritation, or menstrual cramps or pain?
15. Do you have erratic vision or spots before the eyes?
16. Do you suffer from impotence or lack of sexual desire?
    TOTAL "Yes":

If you answered "yes" to one or more questions in the first section, and to two or more in the second section, as well as "yes" to some of the following symptom descriptions, then candida is something you should give attention to:

- Symptoms usually worse on damp days?
- Persistent drowsiness?
- Lack of coordination?
- Headaches?
- Mood swings?
- Loss of balance?
- Rashes?
- Mucus in stools?
- Belching and gas?

- Bad breath?
- Dry mouth or throat?
- Postnasal drip?
- Nasal itching and/or congestion?
- Nervous irritability?
- Tightness in chest?
- Ear sensitivity or fluid in ears?
- Heartburn and indigestion?

SUMMARY, AND A LEADING RESEARCHER'S OPINIONS

There is every reason to believe that candida is a rampant problem in modern society. It has been let loose by the widespread use of pharmaceutical drugs as well as by a dietary pattern that favors the proliferation of the yeast. The number and variety of possible consequences is mind-boggling and deserves the attention of everyone in the healing professions. Yet candida is a condition that is completely amenable to self-assessment and self-help, and the information provided in subsequent chapters should facilitate improvement in most cases in which candida is the main culprit, or where it is a part of the cause of symptoms.

So, you might well ask, if candida represents such a huge problem, and if it can often be controlled by relatively low-tech methods such as those described in this book, then why are these approaches not being actively promoted by medical practitioners?

I do not have a definitive answer to this question, but I think it is useful to share the views of a leading American expert, Dr. Jack Sobel, Dean of the Wayne State University

School of Medicine, where he is also professor of immunology and microbiology, and obstetrics and gynecology. Dr. Sobel has served as a consultant to the U.S. Centers for Disease Control, and has been consistently named a "Top Doctor" since 1995, a "Best Doctor in America" since 1998, and a "Super Doctor" since 2011. In a study published in 1998 he summarizes the major factors in the current candida epidemic as: genetics, pregnancy, diabetes, high-estrogen oral contraceptives, steroid medications (e.g. cortisone), antibiotic usage, intrauterine device usage, frequent sexual intercourse, immunosuppression (as in HIV infection), and sometimes a high-sugar diet.

There are clearly some areas in Dr. Sobel's list of contributing factors that can be controlled: less sugar, safe sex (thereby avoiding IUDs or the pill), and (as far as possible without being reckless) avoiding cortisone, hormone-replacement therapy, antibiotics, and steroid medications. As for those factors on his list that cannot be easily controlled (pregnancy and serious underlying health problems), it is still possible to work at maintaining optimal health by means of diet, exercise, stress reduction, and use of probiotics.

But can probiotics really control yeast? Consider the following conclusions, from a 2010 study by Ehrström et al.:

> This double-blind, placebo controlled clinical study showed the first evidence that a short (five days) period of probiotic supplementation can lead to vaginal colonization of the exogenous lactobacilli for up to six months. . . . So far, all vaginitis and vaginosis treatments have solely been focused on attacking the disproportionately developed bacteria but have not addressed

the restoration of a vaginal acidic environment, i.e., the environment allowing the proliferation of lactic acid–producing *Bacillus acidophilus.*

In other words, women with vaginal candidiasis can "override" a yeast overgrowth rapidly and effectively—and most important, lastingly—by supplementing with friendly bacteria. See chapter 5 for a more detailed discussion of probiotics and other helpful supplements.

LITERATURE

CDC. "Antibiotic Resistance Threats in the United States, 2013: Fluconazole-Resistant *Candida.*" www.cdc.gov/drugresistance/threat-report-2013/pdf/ar-threats-2013-508.pdf.

Cleveland, A. A., L. H. Harrison, M. M. Farley, R. Hollick, B. Stein, T. M. Chiller, S. R. Lockhart, and B. J. Park. "Declining Incidence of candidemia and the shifting epidemiology of *Candida* resistance in two U.S. metropolitan areas, 2008–2013: Results from population-based surveillance." *PLoS One* 10, no. 3 (2015).

Dismukes, W. E., J. S. Wade, J. Y. Lee, B. K. Dockery, and J. D. Hain. "A randomized, double-blind trial of nystatin therapy for the candidiasis hypersensitivity syndrome." *New England Journal of Medicine* 323, no. 25 (1990): 1717–23.

Doyle, C., W. A. Swain, H. A. Ewald, C. L. Cook, and P. W. Ewald. "Sexually transmitted pathogens, depression, and other manifestations associated with premenstrual syndrome." *Human Nature* 26, no. 3 (2015): 277–91.

Ehrström, S., K. Daroczy, E. Rylander, C. Samuelsson, U. Johannesson, B. Anzén, and C. Påhlson. "Lactic acid bacteria colonization and clinical outcome after probiotic supplementation in conventionally treated bacterial vaginosis and vulvovaginal candidiasis." *Microbes and Infection* 12, no. 10 (2010): 691–99.

Finlay, Sue. "A Disease Doctors Don't Recognise." *Observer,* June 1, 1986.

Hidalgo, J. A., and J. A. Vazquez. "Candidiasis," edited by M. S. Bronze, 2014. Available at http://emedicine.medscape.com/article/213853-overview#aw2aab6b2b3aa (accessed June 7, 2016).

Jain, K. K., S. K. Mittal, S. Kumar, and R. K. Gupta. "Imaging features of central nervous system fungal infections." *Neurology India* 55, no. 3 (2007): 241–50.

Lass-Flörl, C., M. P. Diericha, D. Fuchsb, E. Semenitzc, I. Jeneweina, and M. Ledochowskid. "Antifungal activity against *Candida* species of the selective serotonin-reuptake inhibitor sertraline." *Clinical Infectious Diseases* 33 (2001): e135–e136.

Magill, S. S., J. R. Edwards, W. Bamberg, et al. "Multistate point-prevalence survey of health care-associated infections." *New England Journal of Medicine* 370, no. 13 (2014): 1198–208.

Mikulska, M., V. D. Bono, S. Ratto, and C. Viscoli. "Occurrence, presentation and treatment of candidemia." *Expert Review of Clinical Immunology* 8, no. 8 (2012): 755–65.

Murray, Michael T., and Joeseph E. Pizzorno. *The Encyclopedia of Natural Medicine.* 3rd ed. New York: Atria, 2012.

Pfaller, M. A., and D. J. Diekema. "Epidemiology of invasive candidiasis: A persistent public health problem." *Clinical Microbiology Reviews* 20, no. 1 (2007): 133–63.

Sobel, J. D. "Recurrent vulvovaginal candidiasis." *American Journal of Obstetrics and Gynecology* 214, no. 1 (2016): 15–21.

———, S. Faro, R. W. Force, B. Foxman, W. J. Ledger, P. R. Nyirjesy, et al. "Vulvovaginal candidiasis: Epidemiologic, diagnostic, and therapeutic considerations." *American Journal of Obstetrics and Gynecology* 178, no. 2 (1998): 203–11.

Truss, C. Orion. "Restoration of immunological competence to *Candida albicans.*" *Journal of Orthmolecular Psychiatry* 9, no. 4 (1980): 287–301.

Watson, C., et al. "Premenstrual vaginal colonization of *Candida* and symptoms of vaginitis." *Journal of Medical Microbiology* 61(Pt 11) (2012): 1580–83.

Wisplinghoff, H., T. Bischoff, S. M. Tallent, H. Seifert, R. P. Wenzel, and M. B. Edmond. "Nosocomial bloodstream infections in U.S. hospitals: Analysis of 24,179 cases from a prospective nationwide surveillance study." *Clinical and Infectious Diseases* 39, no. 3 (2004): 309–17.

CHAPTER 5

Controlling Candida Naturally

🍂

Supplements, Probiotics, and Herbal Extracts

In this chapter we will review a range of tactics that may be helpful to employ if the digestive tract has become inflamed or irritated by the activity of candida. If after reading the information in the past four chapters and then answering the questionnaire in the previous chapter it seems to you that candida is a likely cause of your condition, then you can test this hypothesis by means of adopting an anticandida program. If this succeeds in making a major improvement in your health by virtue of its controlling candida and improving your symptom picture, then you will have proved your assumption to be correct. In his book *The Yeast Connection,* Dr. William G. Crook calls this approach a "therapeutic trial." It is really the only way of being absolutely sure, since there is as yet no way of definitively establishing whether candida is clinically involved in producing your symptoms by any laboratory tests.

This can be a stumbling block for people who insist on concrete proof that candida is the culprit. Yet all we can do is look at the current big picture of your health and add to this a review of your history. If it looks like a candida picture, then there really is no other choice than to introduce anticandida measures. If your fluid discharges, tissues, or excreta were cultured, the results would almost inevitably display candida's presence somewhere in your body, which would not prove or disprove anything as far as your symptoms are concerned, since a positive test result could also be obtained from almost every adult both with and without symptoms. It is only by looking at known and suspected patterns and symptoms of candida activity that we can guess its active presence (as opposed to its benign presence if your immune system and intestinal flora are keeping it under control). Thus the only real proof is in treatment results. If you are better after controlling candida, then you will know that you assumed correctly and that your program is correct. And at the very least you will have reformed your dietary habits and consumed some beneficial vitamins and other supplements, as well as strengthened your immune system's ability to combat all its adversaries.

It is reasonable to question whether it is really necessary to attack candida when it is obviously active in a local region (oral or vaginal thrush, for example) with an approach that is aimed at the intestinal tract. Fortunately, there is now ample evidence that this is the right way to tackle the problem. Researchers writing in the *American Journal of Obstetrics and Gynecology* detailed their findings in a study that involved 258 women with serious vulvovaginal candidiasis, who were all assessed positive for intestinal candida activity. The patients were divided into two groups, one of which received antifungal medication both by mouth (for the intestines) and vaginally. The other group used antifungal medication locally in the vagina and additionally took a placebo. The medication was used for just one week, and the women were reassessed after one week, three weeks, and seven weeks. The results showed that 88 percent of those receiving both the digestive-tract and local antifungal treatment were clear of candida overgrowth, as opposed to the group that had intravaginal therapy alone, which had a 75 percent success rate. While this shows that significant, although not massive, improvements are achieved when both the local (vaginal) and the intestinal candida are addressed, the study also showed that recurrence of candida overgrowth is lessened among those women who take the dual approach. What this means is that if you treat local thrush and/or yeast-induced vaginitis locally, without treating the overgrowth in the intestinal tract, you will probably improve, but there will be an equal probability of a rapid recurrence. If the intestinal overgrowth is treated in addition to the local symptoms, however, recurrence becomes far less likely.

Controlling candida involves a multipronged approach:

1. Avoid those factors that encourage yeast overgrowth, including, wherever possible, steroid and antibiotic medications.
2. Use natural antifungal products such as caprylic acid, berberine, garlic, and oregano oil, as well as nutrients such as biotin, which retard yeast from changing to its fungal form.
3. Stick to an anticandida dietary pattern (described later in this chapter), and absolutely avoid all sugar and refined carbohydrates.

4. Improve the health of the intestines, especially in relation to permeability ("leaky gut"), and recolonize the intestines with friendly bacteria (including the use of prebiotics and probiotics as described in this chapter).

5. Improve detoxification functions, specifically those involving the liver.

6. Enhance overall immune function by making changes in lifestyle and diet, and consider using vitamin/mineral and herbal supplementation.

These aspects of the anticandida program are described in this chapter, along with some specialized advice for local (oral and vaginal) yeast problems. In chapter 6 we'll take a look at diet and discuss how to "starve" yeast of its favorite sustenance, depriving it of its ability to proliferate. We'll talk about which foods to avoid that might provoke allergic-type reactions in those who have become yeast-sensitive as a result of candida overgrowth.

The sequence in which the different elements of an anticandida program are introduced may need to vary, depending on the particular requirements of each person. For example, sometimes it is necessary to spend some weeks supporting liver function so that it will be better able to handle the detoxification role it plays as yeast dies off. Or the digestive tract might require attention before anything else is attempted. Whatever sequence is adopted, the specific needs of the individual person must be the deciding factors as to the details of each aspect of the whole program.

AVOID ANYTHING
THAT SUPPORTS CANDIDA

Unless absolutely necessary, the contraceptive pill, hormone-replacement therapy, and steroid medications (such as cortisone) and antibiotics should be completely avoided for the duration of the anticandida program.

Dietary recommendations that support a healthy intestinal ecology are described fully in the next chapter, however, briefly here, the basic strategy should be to avoid foods that feed the yeast, such as sugar and refined carbohydrates (white-flour products, for example). A high-fat intake and high stress levels, which can create an acidic environment in the digestive system, should also be avoided. Pre- and probiotics are discussed later in this chapter, including advice on how to encourage healthier, "friendly" bacteria. The bottom line is: the healthier your intestinal tract, the less chance candida has of invading and colonizing territory.

USE NATURAL
ANTIFUNGAL PRODUCTS

Just as different bacterial strains are resistant to particular antibiotics, so different strains of candida can be more or less vulnerable to different herbal products and drugs. Recommended herbal extracts include caprylic acid, garlic, berberine, Kolorex (a natural candida remedy based on the ancient New Zealand herb horopito), oregano oil, and pau d'arco. Other products are sometimes used, but the selection that follows includes those that I have found most useful over many years of treating chronic candidiasis.

Caution: The herbal/plant extracts below should not be taken by pregnant or nursing women.

Caprylic Acid

This extract of the coconut palm destroys candida effectively. Caprylic acid mimics the fatty acids produced by normal bowel flora, which are a major factor in the body's control over candida. It has been successfully used in a time-release form that allows its release in the lower intestinal tract, as a treatment for those with severe intestinal candida. However, if not used in a time-release form, caprylic acid is less effective, as it is absorbed in the upper intestinal region. Caprylic acid is preferable over common antifungal drugs such as nystatin, which is itself yeast-based. Research at Wayne State University in Detroit shows that when nystatin treatment is stopped, even more colonies of yeast develop than were present before its use. Caprylic acid has no such rebound effect once you stop using it after candida is under control.

Caprylic acid is now widely available at health-food stores and some pharmacies. The suggested dosage varies, but good results have been obtained by using 1000 to 2000 mg of time-release capsules three times a day with meals. It is an alternative to using oil of oregano.

Undecylenic Acid (Calcium Undecylenate)

This is a safe and useful broad-spectrum antifungal, a fatty acid extracted from castor bean oil. Its action is similar to, and usually more potent than, that of caprylic acid. Undecylenic acid is a major ingredient of combination formulations that also contain caprylic acid and other antifungals such as pau d'arco. As with caprylic acid, it is important to use time-release capsules of undecylenic acid to avoid it being absorbed too high up in the gastrointestinal tract, thereby not reaching its targets.

Garlic

Garlic has been the subject of worldwide research. Studies have proved its long-reputed antimicrobial and antifungal properties, as well as its action against *Salmonella typhimurium* and *Escherichia coli,* two extremely active microorganisms. Garlic is extremely effective against yeast and fungi. It can easily be incorporated into one's diet, used as a seasoning on cooked vegetables, or crushed into salads. Or you can simply eat the raw cloves or use it with fish or poultry as many Greeks do. The suggested dosage is 400 to 600 mg three times a day with food (supplements should contain approximately 4000 mcg of allicin per capsule) or one clove of fresh garlic daily.

Berberine

Berberine is a quaternary ammonium salt from the proto-berberine group of isoquinoline alkaloids. It is found in such plants as *Berberis aquifolium* (Oregon grape), *Berberis vulgaris* (barberry), *Berberis aristata* (tree turmeric), *Hydrastis canadensis* (goldenseal), *Xanthorhiza simplicissima* (yellowroot), *Phellodendron amurense* (Amur cork tree), *Coptis chinensis* (Chinese goldthread), *Tinospora cordifolia* (heart-leaved moonseed), *Argemone mexicana* (prickly poppy), and *Eschscholzia californica* (California poppy).

Berberine has a wide spectrum of antibiotic activity against bacteria, protozoa, and fungi. Berberine's action against *Candida albicans* has been shown to be more powerful than most medical drugs commonly used for these pathogens.

It has been shown to deactivate not only *Candida albicans* but ten other fungal species.

Berberine's action against candida prevents its overgrowth after antibiotic use and also helps to repopulate the gut with friendly bacteria. In addition to being able to destroy bacteria, yeasts, and viruses, berberine is also an antidiarrhea agent with immune-enhancing capabilities.

Suggested dosages include three different options:

- 1 to 2 g of dried bark or root of *Berberis vulgaris* or *Hydrastis canadensis* (powdered or as a tea) three times daily; or
- 1 to 1½ teaspoons (4 to 6 ml) of a tincture of either of these plants (diluted 1:5), three times daily; or
- ¼ to ½ teaspoon of a fluid extract of either of these plants, three times daily.

Echinacea angustifolia (Purple Coneflower)

Purple coneflower, a North American plant species in the sunflower family, is a Native American herb that offers benefits similar to those of berberine in that it is a powerful antiviral and antifungal agent and an immune-system enhancer. Some products combine echinacea, hydrastis, and berberine together with other immune-enhancing nutrients, such as zinc and vitamin C.

The dosage recommendations for encapsulated products is 750 to 1500 mg daily in divided doses.

Horopito

The New Zealand plant of the *Pseudowintera* genus, commonly known as horopito, is the principal ingredient of

Kolorex. This very slow-growing shrub has leaves that contain a strong antifungal agent, polygodial, which is particularly effective against *Candida albicans*. Studies have found that polygodial compares favorably with the powerful pharmaceutical antifungal amphotericin B. A study that tested eighty-two women with recurring vulvovaginal candidiasis over a period of twelve months found that horopito is "a natural antifungal phytocompound [that] proves to be as good as itraconazole in the maintenance treatment of RVVC [recurring vulvo-vaginal candidiasis]."

The recommended dosage is one capsule containing approximately 350 mg daily of polygodial taken at the same time as 450 mg of anise seed (one capsule of each).

Saccharomyces boulardii

Saccharomyces boulardii is a powerful antifungal yeast derived from the lychee and mangosteen fruit, and it is used as a probiotic to introduce friendly bacteria. It is recommended for all anticandida programs. Recommended dose is 250 mg twice daily. It should be noted, however, that in some severely immunocompromised individuals, *S. boulardii* has been associated with fungemia, or localized infection, which may be fatal.

Grape Seed Extract

Grape seed extract is a proven antibacterial, antiviral, antiparasitic, and antifungal agent, with a high success rate for eliminating candida. In one study it was found that "GSE alone inhibited growth of *C. albicans* yeast cells, and that in a murine model of disseminated candidiasis, mice groups given GSE before intravenous inoculation with the yeast cells survived longer than diluent-received (control) mice groups (P<0.05). This GSE antifungal effect was dose-dependent."

As part of an anticandida program between 100 and 200 mg daily is recommended.

Oil of Oregano

The essential oil of oregano contains powerful antifungal compounds. Side effects are minimal, although allergic reactions to oregano oil can occur, therefore you should stop taking oregano oil if allergic signs or symptoms appear. This is one of the most useful antifungals and is widely available. One study found that "both the oregano and Mexican oregano essential oils showed high levels of antifungal activity against . . . fluconazole-susceptible *C. glabrata*" subjects.

If possible, oregano oil should be taken in an enteric-coated capsule, which delays its release until it reaches the intestinal tract. The recommended dosage is 0.2 to 0.4 ml of an enteric-coated capsule twice a day between meals as an alternative to caprylic acid or calcium undecylenate. Pure oregano oil should only be used following advice from a nutritionist.

Pau d'Arco

The inner bark of a South American tree of the *Tabebuia* genus has a long history of folk use in the treatment of a wide variety of afflictions. Researchers have shown that pau d'arco extracts (containing lapachol) have strong antifungal actions and are particularly effective against *Candida albicans*. Pau d'arco is commonly taken in the form of a tea, consumed several times daily.

Aloe Vera

The juice of this desert plant is a powerful antifungal agent. The healing qualities of aloe vera have been known since Phoenician times. In recent years, attention has been drawn to its usefulness in a range of digestive conditions. Jeffrey Bland, a widely recognized authority in the nutritional medicine field, has demonstrated that the activity of the fresh juice on candida can help sufferers. In a study published in *Preventive Medicine* he says:

> The effect of *Aloe vera* juice supplementation appeared to be that of altering colonic biota. Those subjects that had heavy overgrowth of fecal bacteria and some yeast infection were found to have improved fecal colonization and decreased yeast after the *Aloe vera* juice supplementation. This may indicate that the *Aloe vera* contains an agent or agents which are mycostatic or bacteriostatic or that the improved gastrointestinal function and altered pH of the bowel as it relates to *Aloe vera* juice supplementation sets the stage for different populations of [friendly] bacteria to flourish in the gut.

Aloe vera juice has a similar effect on bacterial and fungal infections of the skin, and it can be applied locally. One or two teaspoonfuls of aloe vera juice in water should be taken twice daily by anyone with candida problems. (Note: once opened, aloe vera juice should be kept refrigerated. The optimum shelf life after opening is about one month.)

Tea Tree Oil

This remarkable extract of the Australian plant *Melaleuca alternifolia* has powerful antifungal properties. Douching daily with a 1 percent solution in water (or, once a week, soaking a tampon into such a solution and inserting it into the vagina as a pessary, leaving it there for no more than twenty-four hours) can be very helpful for vaginitis or cervicitis. This approach is useful whether the cause is candida or trichomonas. Tea tree oil can also be used as a gargle or mouthwash (one drop in a tumbler of water) for oral thrush, or applied directly onto the skin as an ointment. It is somewhat irritating to the skin if used neat as an oil, but there are many products with a 15 percent tea-tree-oil content that are relatively nonirritating.

Chamomile

The plant known as *Matricaria chamomilla* contains antifungal substances in its oil extract. Used as a tea or for topical application, it has soothing qualities similar to pau d'arco.

Tannate Plant Extracts

Plant extracts called tannates (such as the tannin in tea) are powerful antifungal agents. When taken orally, they destroy yeasts selectively, including their spores, without harming the natural flora of the body. There are also formulations for use in the mouth when candida is locally active, and for intravaginal use when thrush is evident. An advantage of using tannates is that they act only in the digestive tract and are not absorbed at all elsewhere, unlike fatty acids, which may be absorbed too high up in the digestive tract unless delivered in suitable time-release capsules.

Additionally, tannates are also useful for detoxifying heavy metals from the body and are therefore suitable for use when mercury toxicity, for example, is a factor in immunosuppression.

Up to six (but usually three) capsules of 600 mg each of tannate products are suggested with every meal for up to eight weeks for chronic candidiasis. Avoid taking tannate tablets on an empty stomach.

Antiparasitic Herb and Plant Extracts

Extracts of citrus (usually grapefruit) seeds have been promoted as safe, natural anticandida and antiparasitic agents. In one Polish study researchers concluded "that 33% grapefruit extract exerts a potent antifungal activity against the yeast-like fungi strains [i.e., candida] and had low activity against dermatophytes and moulds."

Additional antiparasitic herbal assistance is found with berberine (see above) and also *Artemisia annua,* a traditional Chinese herb (not to be confused with *Artemisia absinthum,* a traditional European herb that can be toxic and is illegal in some countries) that is commonly combined with grapefruit seed extract as an antifungal and antiparasitic medicine. A number of safe, antiparasitic herbal combinations are available at health-food stores. Most are effective against both yeasts and parasites, such as combinations of berberine, artemisia, and grapefruit seed extract.

Biotin

Biotin, a water-soluble B vitamin (vitamin B_7), is an important nutrient that combats candida activity when taken with probiotic supplementation. One study showed that biotin inhibits the formation of hyphae, the branching filaments produced by candida species that can penetrate soft tissue (and may cause leaky gut syndrome in the case of intestinal candida).

Biotin deficiency produces a number of skin conditions, including a dermatitis that is characterized by a grayish, dry, flaky appearance. This is accompanied by a lack of appetite, nausea, lassitude, and muscle pain. It is noteworthy that all of these symptoms are also commonly seen when candida proliferates, and it is worth questioning whether the supposed symptoms of biotin deficiency are not at least in part the result of the candida activity brought about by the deficiency.

Egg whites contain a substance called *avidin,* which is capable of combining with biotin, thus neutralizing its usefulness in the body. For this reason, raw egg should not be included in the anticandida diet (although avidin is destroyed by cooking).

Biotin should be taken as a supplement three times daily (between meals) in doses of 350 to 500 mcg, in association with *Lactobacillus acidophilus.*

Olive Oil

Olive oil is a further aid in the prevention of the transformation of candida to its mycelial form. Olive oil contains oleic acid, which acts on the yeast in a similar way as biotin. The recommended amount of olive oil is six teaspoons daily, divided into three doses. This can be included in the meal (added to salad or cooked vegetables), or taken before or after meals as desired. Ensure that the olive oil is virgin, cold-pressed, and organic.

THE ANTICANDIDA DIET

The anticandida diet is the focus of chapter 6. This represents the single most important aspect of the entire anticandida program. In the last thirty years since publication of the first edition of this book, I have been actively teaching people how to follow an anticandida diet, and over the years a significant number of people have informed me that they benefited enormously from the change of diet alone when, for one reason or another (such as economic factors or a lack of availability of specific products), they did not follow the entire program. Depriving yeast of its main food source, sugar, is far and away the most important (and for some people, the most difficult) part of an anticandida protocol.

HEALING THE INTESTINES, REDUCING PERMEABILITY, REPOPULATING WITH FRIENDLY BACTERIA

For friendly bacteria to rapidly recolonize the territory taken over by candida (or other bacteria and yeasts), a number of elements need to be in place: an improved environment, including the right sort of food for these bacteria, or prebiotics; deactivation of the yeast (as described in the previous section on supplementation); healing of the irritated, often inflamed and undesirably permeable mucous membranes to which they need to attach; and a plentiful supply of colonizing organisms. Research suggests that a combination of pre- and probiotics (also known as *symbiotics*) is the ideal approach, and that is what I recommend.

Prebiotics
The way in which the normal flora of the large intestine, bifidobacteria, are nourished has a dramatic effect on how well these bacteria function. Since they perform a number

of important functions, including manufacturing certain vitamins and detoxifying the intestines as well as controlling undesirable bacteria and yeasts from spreading, it is in our best interests to keep them healthy. The functional efficiency of the bifidobacteria is reduced when the diet is rich in animal fats and refined carbohydrates. On the other hand, certain foods known as *prebiotics* can improve their function.

A prebiotic is a nondigestible food ingredient that beneficially affects the host by selectively stimulating the growth and/or activity of one or a limited number of bacteria in the colon, thus improving host health. The beauty of prebiotics is that they specifically help only the friendly bacteria and do not nourish disease-causing organisms. Also, despite being carbohydrate-based, prebiotics are not digested and absorbed and therefore do not increase your weight.

Among the best known of the prebiotics are fructooligosaccharides (FOS), glucooligosaccharides (GOS), and lactosucrose, which have all been shown to be capable of improving the status of the intestinal flora (*B. bifidum* and *L. acidophilus*) after only a short period of time. Many fruits and vegetables contain prebiotics such as FOS, including onions, garlic, bananas, asparagus, leeks, wheat, barley, and Jerusalem artichokes, as well as the blue agave plant. To ensure an intake of prebiotics sufficient to make a difference to the bowel ecology, a great deal of such food needs to be eaten, so supplementing with a concentrated form of FOS, for example, is suggested to boost intake. Concentrated forms exist as liquid extracts or in capsule form and are widely available from health-food stores and pharmacies. Research shows that not less than 4 g and ideally 8 g of FOS should be taken daily to help your friendly bacteria.

An additional boost to the efficient functioning of bifidobacteria and *L. acidophilus* is the presence in the intestine of a nonresident organism, *Lactobacillus bulgaricus,* one of the yogurt-making bacteria, together with *Streptococcus thermophilus.* Thus, supplementation with *L. bulgaricus* will have a prebiotic, or bifidogenic, effect in supporting the function of the normal flora.

Probiotics

As we know, when antibiotics or steroid medications are used, they inevitably destroy a number of the friendly bacteria that inhabit the digestive tract. As well as providing valuable symbiotic (mutually beneficial) contributions to the body, these friendly bacteria also act as a controlling element to stop the spread of candida (as well as other undesirable yeasts and bacteria).

In the average bowel there are huge colonies of microorganisms that can weigh a total of anywhere from three to five pounds. In number, the friendly flora of the bowel exceed the total number of cells in your body. A recent *National Geographic* article on the human microbiome states, "In a new study posted ahead of publication on the bioRxiv website, three scientists led by the Weizmann Institute of Science's Ron Milo find that the average human male is made of 30 trillion cells and contains about 40 trillion bacteria, most of which reside in his digestive tract."

Certainly they are not all helpful or friendly but, when you are healthy, most are. To repopulate the bowel with the more helpful residents requires large quantities of the friendly varieties, mainly *Bifidobacterium bifidum* and *Lactobacillus acidophilus,* which live primarily in the small intestine. When these are recolonized, intruders such as candida are pushed back and often eliminated from the area.

Japanese research has examined the degree of overgrowth of candida as ascertained by the levels found in the feces of leukemia patients receiving drug therapy. Their candida counts were very high before treatment with bifidobacteria supplementation, which reduced levels of candida in some patients from a high of 10,000,000 per gram to 10,000 per gram after treatment. The effectiveness of bifidobacteria in achieving this was seen in all subjects treated, whereas a control group that did not receive bifidobacteria supplementation showed no change at all in their candida levels.

Many researchers report that *Lactobacillus acidophilus* and bifidobacteria actually manufacture substances that retard the growth of candida, and this is borne out when *L. acidophilus* is added to culture dishes in which candida is growing, where its ability to slow and even stop candida growth is evident.

An additional bonus to ingesting bifidobacteria is that it has a uniquely powerful ability to enhance detoxification through the liver as well as detoxifying the intestinal tract itself. Jeffrey Bland says:

> We have been very excited about an alternative therapy for the management of Candida infection which avoids the use of anti-yeast medication (such as nystatin). It is well recognized that a disturbed flora of the GI [gastrointestinal] tract can establish a proper environment for yeast proliferation. By reinoculating [supplementing] the bowel with the proper symbiotic acid-producing bacteria—*Lactobacillus acidophilus* and bifidobacteria— there is a reduction in the compatibility of the intestinal

environment for the yeast proliferation. We have recently used an oral supplement of *Lactobacillus acidophilus*— this has been extremely successful in reducing *Candida albicans* in the intestinal tract. The *Lactobacillus acidophilus* is given as a dry culture.

This approach of using friendly bacteria to repopulate the digestive tract plays a major part in the strategy outlined in this chapter, and it is suitable for anyone with active candida overgrowth. These friendly bacteria (*L. acidophilus* and *B. bifidum*) are among the first of the anticandida supplements you should introduce, together with live, cultured yogurt and/or sour milk with meals (provided you are not allergic to dairy products). These two major probiotic "bacterial friends" will help to control yeast that may have filled the vacant space left behind in the aftermath of antibiotic use (or other factors, such as an imbalanced high-sugar/high-fat diet).

Bacterial cultures intended for supplementation are available in a number of forms, such as powders or in capsules. Cultured milk products (such as live yogurt) containing *L. acidophilus* and *B. bifidum* organisms can also play a part in the anticandida program, although the numbers present in such products are relatively low compared with the high-potency powders and capsules currently available.

How to Take Probiotics

When lactobacilli or bifidobacteria are supplemented, it is vital to ensure that the product you are taking contains not less than one billion viable, active (potentially colony-forming) organisms per gram. This almost always means that the product will need to be kept refrigerated once it has been opened. The potency (number of organisms per gram) needs to be guaranteed at the time of purchase, not at the time of manufacture.

When taking these two organisms therapeutically, as in an anticandida program, they should be taken in equal quantities in water. The amount taken will vary with your condition, but it is usually around 5 to 10 g a day of each in divided doses between meals for a week or more, followed by half that quantity for the duration of the program, which usually runs for three to six months, depending on your progress. A lower, maintenance dose is commonly suggested for long-term use.

A rough guide is that a teaspoonful of powdered probiotic culture is equal to about 2 g, which, depending on potency, equals around two to three billion organisms of each type per teaspoonful.

Powders are usually taken two to three times daily between meals, whereas encapsulated products are usually taken with meals. A supplement of *Lactobacillus bulgaricus* in powder form is also often suggested as an immune-enhancing strategy as well as to improve the colonizing ability of *L. acidophilus* and *B. bifidum*. This should be taken in a dose of around a teaspoonful of powdered culture with each meal. Children under the age of seven should be supplemented with *Bifidobacterium infantis* and not the adult version, and not with *L. acidophilus* unless there has been a recent infection or use of antibiotics, in which case they should be supplemented with both in a ratio of 50:50. A child weighing 77 lbs. (35 kg) should take half the adult quantity of probiotic organisms, and one weighing 44 lbs. (20 kg) or less, a quarter of the adult dose.

PRECAUTIONS WHEN
SUPPLEMENTING WITH PROBIOTICS

- It is suggested that you avoid probiotic products containing additional organisms (other than *L. acidophilus, B. bifidum,* or *L. bulgaricus*), such as *Streptococcus faecium* and *Lactobacillus casei.* This is because the only reason to include these in any mixture is usually a commercial one; there are few dangers, except for a loss of quality and a waste of money.

- Try to obtain specific strains of the organisms, for example, LB-51, a superefficient strain of *L. bulgaricus,* and DDS-1, a well-documented superstrain of *L. acidophilus.*

- Make sure that the container in which the organisms are purchased is made of dark glass, and that there is a guarantee of potency up to an expiration date on the label, and that refrigeration is recommended.

- Avoid liquid probiotic products; stick with powders (best) or capsules. Avoid tablets as well, as the process of manufacturing them destroys much of the potential of the organisms to colonize.

- If possible, ensure (by asking the retailer or manufacturer) that the product was not centrifuged, a process whereby the organisms are separated from the supernatant (the "soup" in which they are grown), which is damaging to them and reduces their colonizing potential.

- If you are dairy-sensitive, make sure that the culture was not grown on a dairy base. Many other options are available from the better manufacturers.

- Whenever possible, obtain each organism in a separate container, as they are not compatible with each other when kept together, even if freeze-dried. An exception to this is when the *L. acidophilus* and *B. bifidum* have been separated by a special process of microencapsulation.

- Follow the manufacturer's advice regarding when the product should be taken (at mealtimes or between meals).
- Do not be confused by claims that particular products are "human strains" or "human compatible." All high-quality probiotic products are suitable for human use.

If you follow these recommendations, you will obtain products of a quality appropriate for an anticandida program. Many practitioners suggest waiting for a week or two after commencing an anticandida program before probiotic supplementation. I prefer to start them immediately as they enhance detoxification of the waste products of the yeast, which is dying off, and the sooner recolonization can start, the better. If the gut wall has become inflamed due to candida activity, then recolonization may take longer than is ideal. However, the strategies suggested below can assist in this.

Healing the Intestinal Mucous Membrane

At the same time that prebiotic and probiotic supplementation commences, particular attention should be given to ensuring that the intestinal walls are in a state that will allow recolonization by the friendly bacteria. If candida overgrowth has caused damage to the walls of the intestinal tract, then recolonization will be difficult. There are other dangers as well. Candida damages the intestinal mucosa, which leads to an increase in its permeability, resulting in leaky gut syndrome, which in turn allows large molecules of incompletely digested food protein and yeast byproducts to enter the bloodstream, thus provoking the immune response.

Food intolerances and allergies play a large part in the symptoms experienced by many people suffering from candida overgrowth, and healing the leaky gut is a key element in eliminating these symptoms. Conditions associated with a leaky gut include asthma, ankylosing spondylitis, Crohn's disease, eczema, food allergies, irritable bowel syndrome (IBS), inflammatory joint disease, malabsorption, psoriasis, Reiter's disease, rheumatoid arthritis, schizophrenia, and ulcerative colitis. To allow better attachment locations for friendly bacteria as well as reducing the load on the immune system, paying attention to irritated intestinal mucous membranes is important. Fortunately, there are a number of natural products that can assist in normalizing this damage. These are best used under expert guidance, however—not for reasons of risk, but to ensure that what is being done is the appropriate course of action.

PRODUCTS THAT HEAL INTESTINAL MUCOSA

- L-glutamine, an amino acid that enhances recovery of damaged mucous membranes
- N-Acetyl-glucosamine (NAG), an amino sugar that is a raw material for reconstruction of tissue damage and that both assists recolonization by friendly bacteria and retards candida's ability to adhere to the wall of the intestines
- Rice-bran oil (gamma-oryzanol), a superbly soothing substance that helps in tissue recovery
- Butyric acid, a normal product of friendly bacteria, also found in olive oil, which helps in mucous-membrane healing
- FOS (fructooligosaccharides, already discussed in this

chapter), usually extracted from vegetables such as Jerusalem artichoke, which encourages healing of the gut wall and recolonization by friendly bacteria

These products, available from health-food stores and many pharmacies, may be taken individually or in various combinations.

Additional assistance to the digestive process is often necessary. This is provided by adding enzyme complexes to the list of supplements. As well, ensuring that adequate digestive acids are present in the stomach during digestion is important. This might call for supplementation with hydrochloric acid capsules or, preferably, with herbs that promote the natural production of acids, such as Swedish bitters.

DETOXIFICATION

Toxicity in the intestines creates an unhealthy ecology that usually involves candida activity and increased gut permeability. This condition of microbial imbalance in the gut is summarized in one word: *dysbiosis*.

To help reduce intestinal dysbiosis, the following nutritional strategies are called for:

- Probiotics (for example *L. acidophilus* and *B. bifidum*)
- Prebiotics (fructooligosaccharides, or FOS: 4 to 8 g daily)
- Foods rich in FOS (onions, asparagus, bananas, Jerusalem artichokes, etc.)
- Fiber-rich foods and/or a fiber supplement (at least 40 g daily of linseed or psyllium seeds)
- Avoidance of allergenic foods

- Specific herbs (such as *Hydrastis canadensis,* i.e., goldenseal)
- Regular intake of *Allium sativum* (garlic)

Toxins that derive from a dysbiotic gut are known as *endotoxins* (different from toxins entering the body from outside, called *exotoxins*). The main defense against toxicity is the liver, which undertakes hundreds of different chemical processes to achieve a toxin-free bloodstream. As the main organ of detoxification, the liver filters blood; secretes fat-soluble toxins via the bile (if there is adequate fiber); contains specialized cells (Kupffer cells or macrophages) that literally engulf toxins as well as deactivate larger immune complexes; uses enzymes to take toxins apart (disassemble), and then excretes the toxins in a complicated, two-phase operation that, if out of balance, allows highly reactive toxins to build up.

It is estimated that approximately 25 percent of detoxification occurs in the gut, much of it as a result of probiotic, friendly bacteria activity, while the remainder takes place in the liver (with water-soluble toxins leaving via the kidneys and fat-soluble ones via the bile).

Liver Support

A program of liver support is often needed before starting the anticandida program fully, as the process of detoxification of dying yeast as well as the possible dysbiotic state of the bowel is likely to place enormous demands on liver function. One of the most potent liver-supporting substances is the herb milk thistle (*Silybum marianum*). In a trial involving hundreds of patients with a variety of liver disorders, after eight weeks of supplementation with milk thistle, over 60 percent reported that all symptoms had disappeared (including nausea, pruritus, abdominal distention, anorexia, and fatigue). Liver function tests confirmed improvement, and liver enlargement decreased, while side effects were minimal.

A dose of 120 mg of milk thistle three times daily has been shown to stimulate regeneration of damaged liver cells.

Other liver-protecting herbs include catechin 35, dandelion root (*Taraxacum officinale*), and artichoke leaves (*Cynara scolymus*).

SUPPLEMENTATION FOR IMMUNE SUPPORT

To strengthen the immune system, a number of essential nutrients should be included in the anticandida program. As not all of these may be necessary in every case, it is important to seek guidance from a qualified nutritional expert to make sure that your particular needs are addressed.

Vitamin C

The importance of vitamin C cannot be overemphasized. T cells, which form a major part of our defense system, contain high levels of vitamin C. It has been noted that the lower the vitamin C content of these vital cells, the less efficient their performance in defending the body against intruding organisms or materials, including yeast.

Any stress, whether originating in the emotions or caused by the presence of toxic pollution, infection, or other factors, places increased demands on vitamin C levels in the body. This is a water-soluble vitamin and the body has no stores of it, so a constant supply is needed. Research has shown a fascinating adaptation that takes place when requirements increase because of stress or infection. Under normal conditions, if a person takes more vitamin C than is actually required, a degree of diarrhea is likely to develop. This is well known and is one way of assessing just how much vitamin C you need. If 5 g are taken daily with no resultant diarrhea, then it can be assumed that this amount of vitamin C is needed at that time. If, however, diarrhea develops after ingesting only 2 g daily, but circumstances alter because of infection or stress, then it is possible to increase vitamin C intake to many times 2 g daily without any bowel symptoms at all. When the crisis passes, however, such doses would produce diarrhea, as before. Thus the body, in its wisdom, seems to be able to alter its function to meet particular requirements in this way.

To bolster a deficient immune system as a result of candida overgrowth, the recommended amount of vitamin C to be supplemented (in the absence of any bowel reaction) is 1 to 3 g daily with food.

Arginine

The effects of vitamin C on the T cells depends on the T cells being there to do their work. The thymus gland, which lies below the breastbone, can become relatively inactive, and one of the main nutrients that can enhance its production of T cells is the amino acid arginine.

A dose of 3 g daily for a short period (say a month) will boost thymus activity at the onset of the program, when it is most needed. Take the arginine before retiring, on an empty stomach, with water. Long-term use of arginine at these dosages is not suggested, although there are no known side-effects with doses lower than 20 g daily. Rough, thick-ened skin may develop on the elbows with doses above 20 g daily, but this will disappear when the supplementation is stopped. The reason for suggesting a time limit for the use of arginine is that the thymus may come to depend on such nutritional supplementation when it should be encouraged to return to normal activity by the total program of can-dida suppression. Therefore, take 3 g daily for only the first month of the program.

Note: If you have a history of herpes simplex infection, do not supplement with arginine, because it has also been found to enhance herpes activity (which is countered by another amino acid, lysine).

B Vitamins

To further aid the immune system, increase your intake of certain of the B vitamins. It is important to the program that these are not derived from yeast sources, as anyone with a can-dida problem is likely to have become yeast-sensitive. All the B vitamins are available in synthetic forms, and these, rather than yeast-derived ones, are suggested for candida. They are readily available at good health-food stores and many pharmacies.

The recommended dosages are 20 to 50 mg of vitamin B_6 (pyridoxine), 20 to 50 mcg of vitamin B_{12}, and 20 to 50 mcg of folic acid daily. In addition, vitamin B_5 should be taken to assist in the enhancement of B lymphocytes, especially if there is evidence of allergic reactions or digestive involvement. This should be taken in the form of pantothenate (pantothenic acid), at a dose of 500 mg daily.

Minerals

The minerals zinc, selenium, and magnesium are all commonly implicated in deficient immune-response conditions and should ideally be added to the program. As with the B vitamins, it is important to obtain a nonyeast source of selenium.

Recommended dosages (all to be taken with food) of these minerals are:

* Zinc (as zinc orotate, picolinate, or citrate), 50 mg daily
* Selenium, 50 mcg daily
* Magnesium, 250 to 500 mg daily

Finally, a supply of some of the fat-soluble vitamins is called for in our effort to resuscitate the immune response. This includes a moderate intake of vitamin E (make sure that you buy natural vitamin E, identified by the name D-alpha-tocopherol, rather than D,L-alpha-tocopherol, which is a synthetic form) at a dose of 200 to 400 IU (international units) daily; vitamin A in the form of beta-carotene, in a dose of up to 100,000 IU daily; and oil of evening primrose (vitamin F) in a 500-mg capsule twice daily, or an alternative such as flaxseed oil.

SUMMARY OF ANTICANDIDA AND IMMUNE-ENHANCING SUPPLEMENTS

Bear in mind that whatever is done to enhance immune function and health and to repair the lining of the gut and to recolonize the digestive tract with friendly bacteria, there must always be an antifungal strategy to eliminate the yeast. If you intend to administer the anticandida protocol yourself, then at the very least take either caprylic acid, horopito, garlic, or oregano oil, as well as following the immune-enhancing and probiotic supplementation suggestions found in this chapter, and the recommendations for an anticandida diet found in the next chapter. Most important, anyone with a candida problem is urged to seek advice from a health care practitioner before embarking on an antifungal program, as there are so many individual variables, and self-treating runs the risk of producing disappointing results.

Note: For quantities, see the notes earlier in this chapter or discuss this with a health care professional (naturopath, nutritionist, or pharmacist).

Items below marked +++ are always indicated for candida treatment. All other substances require individualized prescribing by a suitably qualified health care professional.

FOR RECOLONIZATION

- *Lactobacillus acidophilus* and *Bifidobacterium* (at least two billion viable organisms of each daily) +++
- *Saccharomyces boulardii* is recommended for most anticandida programs, particularly if diarrhea is a problem (250 mg twice daily)*
- Biotin (vitamin H) +++
- FOS (at least 8 g daily) +++

---

*Some caution has been urged for those who are immune compromised, although a study conducted in 2015 suggests that *S. boulardii* is perfectly safe even for HIV-treated patients.

ANTIFUNGAL AGENTS (AT LEAST ONE, OR A COMBINATION OF SEVERAL OF THESE, IS ESSENTIAL)

- Garlic
- Aloe vera juice
- Echinacea, hydrastis, and/or berberine
- Pau d'arco
- Polygodial (horopito)
- Caprylic acid
- Oregano oil
- Olive oil
- Tannates
- Chamomile
- *Saccharomyces boulardii*

IMMUNE FUNCTION ENHANCEMENT (AS INDICATED BY HISTORY AND CONDITION)

- Vitamin C
- Vitamin E
- Vitamin A (as beta-carotene)
- Arginine
- Pantothenate (vitamin B_5/pantothenic acid)
- Vitamin B_6 (pyridoxine)
- Vitamin B_{12}
- Folic acid
- Or a high-potency vitamin B-complex capsule (yeast-free, slow release, containing not less than 50 mg each of the major B vitamins)
- Selenium
- Zinc
- Magnesium
- Oil of evening primrose (or other forms of essential fatty

acids, including flaxseed, borage, and blackcurrant seeds, as well as fish oils)

OTHER NUTRIENTS

- Chromium (particularly if there is low blood sugar)
- Iron
- Manganese
- Full-spectrum amino acids
- Nutrient combinations including glutamine, gamma-oryzanol, and N-acetyl glucosamine (NAG) for healing gut mucous membrane
- Liver-support substances, such as milk thistle

To summarize, several strategies are needed at the same time to deal with the problems created by candida. First, we use probiotics and biotin (as well as herbal and other products as discussed) to directly inhibit candida and fight its spread. Other nutrients are used to build up immune function (B and T cells) so that the body can better cope with the invading microorganisms. Therefore, this part of the anticandida program requires taking a large number of supplements, which can be both somewhat expensive and off-putting. Let it be clear, however, that what is at stake is your health. For this reason, there should be no hesitation in grasping this opportunity to fight off the cause of your ill health by whatever safe methods are at hand. The methods being advocated here are safe as well as effective in most cases. It can take time to control candida once it is rampant, and six months should be seen as the minimum length of time to maintain this program.

YEAST DIE-OFF

During periods of rapid yeast destruction as the supplementation and dietary program proceeds, the body's organs of elimination (such as the liver) will be called on to detoxify the breakdown products of this process. This can lead to your feeling particularly irritable and nauseated. This reaction is what is known as yeast die-off or burn-off (or Herxheimer's reaction), and it can last anywhere from several days to weeks. The use of beneficial strains of high-potency bifidobacteria, together with the general dietary strategies discussed in this and the next chapter, should minimize this kind of reaction. In any case, do not be tempted to stop the anticandida program when this process becomes evident, as it does not indicate that the program is not working—indeed, quite the contrary. This is a critical stage of the treatment that, if stopped suddenly, can lead to a rebound of candida activity and even greater feelings of ill health. This die-off period does not usually last for more than a week or ten days, by which time, if you've stuck to the guidelines, a gradual improvement should be evident. Total control of the fungus, and therefore eradication of all symptoms, can, however, take many months.

CAUTIONS AND POSSIBLE SIDE EFFECTS

- If you have an eating disorder such as anorexia or bulimia, do not attempt to change your diet radically without expert advice and supervision.
- Expect that yeast die-off is likely, and that it will cause odd symptoms for a week or so.
- There may be changes in bowel habits, and while these should settle down within a few weeks, seek professional

advice if there is prolonged diarrhea or constipation (increased water intake and linseed oil should normally take care of this).

- If symptoms such as palpitations, unusual fatigue, brain fog, unusual muscle and joint discomfort, or a runny nose appear, suspect a food sensitivity and carefully consider anything new in your diet. Use exclusion and rotation (discussed in chapter 6) to identify any suspected foods or substances, which should then be excluded for at least three months.

- Expect that any local yeast-affected areas will become worse for a few days. This includes oral, vaginal, and skin areas. This will calm down on its own, but it can be helped by the use of local treatment methods.

- Do not be surprised if you start to crave certain foods, sugars and starches in particular. This is usually a result of an imbalance in blood-sugar levels due to dietary changes and should settle down in time. If the craving is bothersome or severe, either take expert advice or use one of the following tactics to help balance blood-sugar levels:

  - Take 1 g daily of the amino-acid L-glutamine (between meals) and assess its effect on the craving.
  - Supplement with 3 to 4 g of full-spectrum amino acids between meals, two or three times daily.
  - Take one 200 mcg chromium tablet daily (glucose tolerance factor) to assist in stabilizing blood sugar levels.
  - Eat small portions and often (from the list of appropriate foods found in chapter 6), with snacks between meals and one late at night before bedtime.

LOCAL ORAL
ANTICANDIDA TREATMENT

Research has shown that a number of over-the-counter mouthwashes are extremely effective in controlling oral candida, by up to 80 percent. The most effective products listed by researchers are Corsodyl, Oraldene, and Listerine, with Colgate Peroxyl achieving a reduction of around 40 percent.

In 2009, lemon juice was tested in the treatment of severe oral thrush. When compared with standard treatment involving gentian violet solution, freshly squeezed lemon juice (20 ml juice to 10 ml water) was found to be vastly superior. Recommended dose: rinse the mouth with half of the mixture for five minutes, then spit out. After five minutes repeat the rinse, and then swallow the juice. Several other times a day place drops of lemon juice against affected areas. This routine is usually effective within ten days.

LOCAL VAGINAL
ANTICANDIDA TREATMENT

A number of approaches may be useful for soothing inflamed vaginal tissues during an anticandida treatment. Whichever one is used, it is imperative that a comprehensive antifungal dietary approach is also followed, or a recurrence of thrush or yeast-caused vaginitis will be very likely.

- Using a special soft-tipped disposable applicator, insert a solution of high-potency *L. acidophilus* culture mixed with pure water or, even better, some diluted aloe vera juice. Any of the acidophilus products recommended for dietary use can be used in this way. Another way to achieve this effect is to puncture an acidophilus capsule with several pin-pricks and to insert the capsule deep into the vagina overnight. The acidophilus will leak out of the capsule and inhibit the yeast, and the empty capsule can be expelled by douching (see below). Alternatively, you can mix a teaspoonful of acidophilus powder or the contents of two capsules with live yogurt and insert this into the vagina overnight, although this will be messy. Finally, douching with water containing a teaspoonful of dissolved acidophilus powder will also be effective.

- Aloe vera juice alone (two teaspoonfuls diluted in a half-pint of water) can be used as a douche to relieve itching and burning.
- Tannate extracts are available (from health-food stores) for use as a douche. These combine irreversibly with yeast cells, deactivating them and also preventing their adherence to the walls of the vagina.
- Tea tree oil used as a pessary or diluted in water as a douche is an effective, if slightly irritating at first, antifungal treatment for any vaginitis of yeast origin.
- Diluted vinegar (or lemon juice) douches, on their own or with acidophilus powder added, are useful for soothing irritated vaginal tissues and for acidifying the area. A more acidic environment is supportive of friendly bacteria and makes it more difficult for yeast to adhere to the vaginal walls. Never use vinegar neat on these sensitive tissues.
- Soothing antifungal calendula (marigold) pessaries are available at some health-food outlets.

COLONIC IRRIGATION AND ENEMAS

Colonic irrigation involves the administration of water into the bowels to clear debris from the region and to encourage its health. Sometimes other substances are added, such as garlic extract and acidophilus. Periodic flushes with water coupled with one of these additives can greatly improve the condition of the bowels. Enemas are less effective since they penetrate only a short distance up the intestines, unlike the colonic, which can pass water along the entire length of the large intestine. The technique requires expert skills, and its use in the treatment of candida problems requires additional knowledge. In principle, however, such a treatment is recommended, at least in the early stages of the program.

A caution is given regarding the excessive use of colonic irrigation; if done too frequently, it can actually deplete the normal intestinal flora. Its use should be limited to an actual need, a precise prescription of the number of applications, and, essentially, for reimplantation of friendly organisms as part of the process.

YEAST DESENSITIZATION TO CONTROL CANDIDA

Carefully controlled doses of candida extract may be injected in an attempt to produce an immune-system response, under the supervision of a medically qualified health care professional. Antibodies thus produced by white blood cells can assist in the defense against antigens entering the system because of the yeast. The use of yeast extracts as a "vaccine" of sorts also appears to assist general immune function by helping to balance or regulate aspects the production of "helper" and "suppressor" cells, as discussed in chapter 2.

However, this whole procedure is extremely complicated because although *Candida albicans* is a clearly identifiable strain of yeast, it has many variables. Thus the candida that grows in one person is never exactly the same as that growing in another. This biological individuality applies to yeasts as much as it does to every other living creature, including people. Therefore, injecting the same extract of candida into two different people will not produce the same response, nor is the yeast likely to be the same as that to which the individual is normally exposed, so this is a process of trial and error. Genetic factors may be largely responsible for the different responses of individuals to such treatment, so anticandida desensitization treatments need to be applied by an expert who is able to cope with all the complex variables.

Even should such expertise be available, this approach, with all its possible pitfalls in terms of different reactions, at best can only deal with just one aspect of the problem. It may assist in bolstering the immune system against the byproducts of candida infestation, which is especially desirable for those who are suffering from the type of allergy symptoms mentioned earlier, but it will do little for the local symptoms currently active in the bowels or reproductive system. Only the harmful effects of candida that are mediated by the bloodstream will be helped by this method. Valuable as that may be, it would leave much of the underlying condition untouched and would still require a program involving an anticandida diet and supplements to control its spread and feeding.

Dr. Truss cautions that this type of "vaccination" program is contraindicated in people suffering from autoimmune conditions, including rheumatoid arthritis. Stimulation of the immune response in someone who is being attacked by his or her own immune system would only lead to aggravation of the condition.

CONVENTIONAL MEDICAL ANTIFUNGAL STRATEGIES

Let me say from the outset that the following is provided purely for information purposes. I do not recommend the conventional medical approach to controlling candida for a variety of reasons, many already discussed. This is because the orthodox medical treatment of fungal infection such as candida involves the use of antifungal antibiotics such as nystatin. This drug is active against a wide range of yeasts and yeastlike fungi, including candida, and comes in a variety of forms—as a liquid for use in the mouth; as tablets for use in treating candida in the intestinal tract; as suppositories for use in the vagina; and as creams, ointments, and powders for the treatment of surface areas such as the skin and nails.

There are a number of commonly used antifungal drugs (as mentioned in chapter 2) that have a number of drawbacks compared to the safer, natural substances discussed in this book.

Nystatin: No less an authority than Dr. William Crook, whose book *The Yeast Connection* has done so much to encourage awareness of the damage candidiasis can cause, has said that nystatin is safe and effective. It's true, nystatin is lethal to yeast cells upon contact. However, getting them into contact with the drug is not always easy, especially if they are deep in the bowels. Also, nystatin passing through the bowels will kill all surface yeasts but none that are embedded deeper into the walls of the intestine. It seems likely that where the gut wall has been damaged by yeast (increased permeability, or leaky gut syndrome), some of the drug may enter the bloodstream with unpredictable results.

Diflucan (fluconazole): This expensive drug requires lengthy use to have any noticeable effects. The more common side effects of this drug include nausea, headache, skin rash, vomiting, abdominal pain, and diarrhea. In some cases, fluconazole can cause serious side effects. These can include liver failure and severe rash.

Ketoconazole: This antifungal drug causes damage to the liver as a result of its easy access to the bloodstream from the intestinal tract.

In medical settings when these drugs are prescribed it is rarely the case that they are recommended along with a comprehensive antifungal dietary and supplement approach to encourage a healthier digestive tract and immune system. In fact, none of these drugs are even necessary, since the methods outlined in this book are safer and of proven efficacy over the long term. If a condition such as candida has become so widespread as to cause a problem, then it is vital that the immune system and bowel flora, which should be controlling the situation, are revitalized. Reliance on nystatin or any other drug will leave your immune system debilitated, except that there will be, over a period of time, fewer yeast byproducts entering the bloodstream to challenge the immune system. This allows the immune system to revive gradually. There is certainly no objection to nystatin being employed if the condition is severe enough to warrant it, but this should only be done in combination with the sort of multipronged approach outlined in this book. Otherwise, there will be only short-term gains, and the condition will most certainly recur.

By relying on a supplementation program as outlined here, together with the dietary guidelines in chapter 6, it is possible to not only control candida but to improve your general well-being dramatically. This is something no drug can achieve, whether it produces side effects or not.

Next we will focus on the importance of a combined attack on candida that includes starving this persistent fungus of its main source of sustenance—sugar.

LITERATURE

Akpan, A., and R. Morgan. "Oral candidiasis." *Postgraduate Medical Journal* 78, no. 922 (2002): 455–59.

Albrecht, M., H. Frerick, U. Kuhn, and A. Strengehesse. "Therapy of toxic liver-disease with Legalon (R)." [Ger]. *Zeitschrift fur Klinische Medizin* 47, no. 2 (1992): 87–92.

Astegiano, M., R. Pellicano, E. Terzi, et al. "Treatment of irritable bowel syndrome: A case control experience." *Minerva Gastroenterologica e Dietologica* 52, no. 4 (2006): 359–63.

Bahmani, M., H. Shirzad, S. Rafieian, and M. Rafieian-Kopaei. "*Silybum marianum:* Beyond hepatoprotection." *Journal of Evidence-Based Complementary and Alternative Medicine* 20, no. 4 (2015): 292–301.

Barnes, J., L. A. Anderson, S. Gibbons, and J. D. Phillipson. "Echinacea species (*Echinacea angustifolia* [DC.] Hell., *Echinacea pallida* [Nutt.] Nutt., *Echinacea purpurea* [L.] Moench): A review of their chemistry, pharmacology and clinical properties." *Journal of Pharmacy and Pharmacology* 57, no. 8 (2005): 929–54.

Bauer, R. "New knowledge regarding the effect and effectiveness of *Echinacea purpurea* extracts." *Wiener Medizinische Wochenschrift* 152, nos. 15–16 (2002): 407–11.

Bland, Jeffrey. "*Candida albicans:* An Unsuspected Problem." Resource Monograph, *Nutritional Biochemistry,* University of Puget Sound, Tacoma, Wa., 1984.

———. "Effect of orally consumed aloe vera juice on gastrointestinal function in normal humans." *Preventive Medicine,* March-April, 1985. Linus Pauling Institute of Science and Medicine, Palo Alto, Calif.

Bruzzese, E., M. Volpicelli, M. Squaglia, et al. "Impact of prebiotics on human health." *Digestive and Liver Disease* 38, suppl. 2 (2006): S283–87.

Casella, S., M. Leonardi, B. Melai, F. Fratini, and L. Pistelli. "The role of diallyl sulfides and dipropyl sulfides in the in vitro antimicrobial activity of the essential oil of garlic, *Allium sativum* L., and leek, *Allium porrum* L." *Phytotherapy Research* 27, no. 3 (2013): 380–83.

Chopra, V., F. Marotta, A. Kumari, M. P. Bishier, F. He, N. Zerbinati, C. Agarwal, et al. "Prophylactic strategies in recurrent vulvovaginal candidiasis: A 2-year study testing a phytonutrient vs itraconazole." *Journal of Biological Regulators and Homeostatic Agents* 27, no. 3 (2013): 875–82.

Ciebiada-Adamiec, A., E. Małafiej, and I. Ciebiada. "Inhibitory effect of nicotinamide on enzymatic activity of selected fungal strains causing skin infection." *Mycoses* 53, no. 3 (2010): 204–7.

Crook, William G. *The Yeast Connection: A Medical Breakthrough.* New York: Vintage, 1986.

———, Hyla Cass, and Elizabeth B. Crook. *The Yeast Connection and Women's Health.* Jackson, Tenn.: Professional Books, 2012.

Cruz, I., J. J. Cheetham, J. T. Arnason, J. E. Yack, and M. L. Smith. "Alkamides from *Echinacea* disrupt the fungal cell wall-membrane complex." *Phytomedicine* 21, no 4 (2014): 435–42.

Del Piano, M., L. Morelli, G. Strozzi, et al. "Probiotics: From research to consumer." *Digestive and Liver Disease* 38 (2006): S248–55.

Dinleyici, E. C., A. Kara, N. Dalgic, et al. "*Saccharomyces boulardii* CNCM I-745 reduces the duration of diarrhoea, length of emergency care and hospital stay in children with acute diarrhoea." *Beneficial Microbes* 6, no. 4 (2015): 415–21.

Doddanna, S. J., S. Patel, M. A. Sundarrao, and R. S. Veerabhadrappa. "Antimicrobial activity of plant extracts on *Candida albicans:* An in vitro study." *Indian Journal of Dental Research* 24, no. 4 (2013): 401–5.

Gibson, G. "Understanding prebiotics in infant and childhood nutrition." *Journal of Family Health Care* 16, no. 4 (2006): 119–22.

Gordillo, M. A., N. Obradors, J. L. Montesinos, et al. "Stability studies and effect of the initial oleic acid concentration on lipase production by *Candida rugosa*." *Applied Microbiology and Biotechnology* 43, no. 1 (1995): 38–41.

Greshko, M. "How many cells are in the human body—and how many microbes?" *National Geographic,* January 13, 2016. Available at http://news.nationalgeographic.com/2016/01/160111-microbiome-estimate-count-ratio-human-health-science (accessed June 8, 2016).

Hammer, K. A., C. F. Carson, and T. V. Riley. "Antifungal effects of *Melaleuca alternifolia* (tea tree) oil and its components on *Candida albicans, Candida glabrata* and *Saccharomyces cerevisiae*." *Journal of Antimicrobial Chemotherapy* 53, no. 6 (2014): 1081–85.

Han, Y. "Synergic effect of grape seed extract with amphotericin B against disseminated candidiasis due to *Candida albicans*." *Phytomedicine* 14, no. 11 (2007): 733–38.

Höfling, J. F., P. C. Anibal, G. A. Obando-Pereda, I. A. Peixoto, V. F. Furletti, M. A. Foglio, and R. B. Gonçalves. "Antimicrobial potential of some plant extracts against *Candida* species." *Brazilian Journal of Biology* 70, no. 4 (2010): 1065–68.

Hossain, F., P. Follett, K. Vu Dang, M. Harich, S. Salmieri, and M. Lacroix. "Evidence for synergistic activity of plant-derived essential oils against fungal pathogens of food." *Food Microbiology* 53, pt. B (2016): 24–30.

Jackson, D. N., L. Yang, S. Wu, E. J. Kennelly, and P. N. Lipke. "Garcinia xanthochymus benzophenones promote hyphal apoptosis and potentiate activity of fluconazole against *Candida albicans* biofilms." *Antimicrobial Agents and Chemotherapy* 59, no. 10 (2015): 6032–38.

Kageyama, T., Y. Nakano, and T. Tomoda. "Comparative study on oral administration of some *Bifidobacterium* preparations." *Medicine and Biology* 115 (1987): 65–68.

———, T. Tomoda, and Y. Nakano. "The effect of *Bifidobacterium* administration in patients with leukemia." *Bifidobacteria Microflora* 3 (1984): 29–33.

Kelesidis, T., and C. Pothoulakis. "Efficacy and safety of the probiotic *Saccharomyces boulardii* for the prevention and therapy of gastrointestinal disorders." *Therapeutic Advances in Gastroenterology* 5 (2012): 111–25.

Krajewska-Kułak, E., C. Lukaszuk, and W. Niczyporuk. "Effects of 33% grapefruit extract on the growth of the yeast-like fungi, dermatopytes and moulds." *Wiadomosci Parazytologiczne* 47, no. 4 (2001): 845–49.

Kumari, A., M. P. Bishier, Y. Naito, A. Sharma, U. Solimene, S. Jain, H. Yadava, E. Minelli, C. Tomella, and F. Marotta. "Protective effect of an oral natural phytonutrient in recurrent vulvovaginal candidiasis: A 12-month study." *Journal of Biological Regulators and Homeostatic Agents* 25, no. 4 (2011): 543–51.

Li, L. P., W. Liu, H. Liu, F. Zhu, Z. da Zhang, H. Shen, Z. Xu, et al. "Synergistic antifungal activity of berberine derivative B-7b and fluconazole." *PLoS One* 10, no. 5 (2015).

Lopetuso, L. R., F. Scaldaferri, G. Bruno, V. Petito, F. Franceschi, and A. Gasbarrini. "The therapeutic management of gut barrier leaking: The emerging role for mucosal barrier protectors." *European Review for Medical and Pharmacological Sciences* 19, no. 6 (2015): 1068–76.

Ludovico, Abenavoli, Raffaele Capasso, Matasa Milic, and Francesco Capasso. "Milk thistle in liver diseases: Past, present, future." *Phytotherapy Research* 24, no. 10 (2010): 1423–32.

McCallion, R. F., A. L. Cole, J. R. Walker, J. W. Blunt, and H. H. Munro. "Antibiotic substances from New Zealand plants. II. Polygodial, an anti-Candida agent from *Pseudowintera colorata*." *Planta Medica* 44, no. 3 (1982): 134–38.

Mekonnen, A., B. Yitayew, A. Tesema, and S. Taddese. "In vitro antimicrobial activity of essential oil of *Thymus schimperi, Matricaria chamomilla, Eucalyptus globulus,* and *Rosmarinus officinalis*." *International Journal of Microbiology* (2016). doi: 10.1155/2016/9545693.

Mir-Rashed, N., I. Cruz, M. Jessulat, M. Dumontier, C. Chesnais, J. Ng, V. T. Amiguet, A. Golshani, J. T. Arnason, and M. L. Smith. "Disruption of fungal cell wall by antifungal *Echinacea* extracts." *Medical Mycology* 48, no. 7 (2010): 949–58.

Nystatin Multicenter Study Group. "Therapy of candidal vaginitis: The effect of eliminating intestinal Candida." *American Journal of Obstetrics and Gynecology* 155, no. 3 (1986): 651–55.

Ota, C., C. Unterkircher, V. Fantinato, and M. T. Shimizu. "Antifungal activity of propolis on different species of *Candida*." *Mycoses* 44, nos. 9–10 (2001): 375–78.

Park, K. S., K. C. Kang, J. H. Kim, D. J. Adams, T. N. Johng, and Y. K. Paik. "Differential inhibitory effects of protoberberines on sterol and chitin biosyntheses in *Candida albicans*." *Journal of Antimicrobial Chemotherapy* 43, no. 5 (1999): 667–74.

Picard, C. J. Fioramonti, A. Francois, T. Robinson, F. Neant, and C. Matuchansky. "Review article: Bifidobacteria as probiotic agents—physiological effects and clinical benefits." *Alimentary Pharmacology and Therapeutics* 22, no. 6 (2005): 495–512.

Ramage, G., et al. "Commercial mouthwashes are more effective than azole antifungals against *Candida albicans* biofilms in vitro." *Oral Surgery, Oral Medicine, Oral Pathology, Oral Radiology, and Endodontology* 111, no. 4 (2011): 456–60.

Salama, A. A., M. AbouLaila, M. A. Terkawi, A. Mousa, A. El-Sify, M. Allaam, A. Zaghawa, N. Yokoyama, and I. Igarashi. "Inhibitory effect of allicin on the growth of *Babesia* and *Theileria* equi parasites." *Parasitology Research* 113, no. 1 (2014): 275–83.

Salmi, H. A., and S. Sarna. "Effect of silymarin on chemical, functional, and morphological alterations of the liver: A double-blind controlled study." *Scandinavian Journal of Gastroenterology* 17, no. 4 (1982): 517–21.

Santino, I., A. Alari, S. Bono, E. Teti, M. Marangi, A. Bernardini, L. Magrini, S. Di Somma, and A. Teggi. "Saccharomyces cerevisiae fungemia, a possible consequence of the treatment of Clostridium difficile colitis with a probioticum. *International Journal of Immunopathological Pharmacology* 27, no. 1 (2014): 143–46.

Shetty, S., B. Thomas, V. Shetty, R. Bhandary, and R. M. Shetty. "An in-vitro evaluation of the efficacy of garlic extract as an antimicrobial agent on periodontal pathogens: A microbiological study." *Ayu* 34, no. 4 (2013): 445–51.

Soares, I. H., É. S. Loreto, L. Rossato, D. N. Mario, T. P. Venturini, F. Baldissera, J. M. Santurio, and S. H. Alves. "In vitro activity of essential oils extracted from condiments against fluconazole-resistant and -sensitive *Candida glabrata.*" *Journal de Mycologie Médicale* 25, no. 3 (2015): 213–17.

Sobel, Jack D. "Recurrent vulvovaginal candidiasis." *American Journal of Obstetrics and Gynecology* 214, no. 1 (2016): 15–21.

Ulusoy, S., G. Ozkan, F. B. Yucesan, Ş. Ersöz, A. Orem, M. Alkanat, E. Yuluğ, K. Kaynar, and S. Al. "Anti-apoptotic and anti-oxidant effects of grape seed proanthocyanidin extract in preventing cyclosporine A-induced nephropathy." *Nephrology* 17, no. 4 (2012): 372–79.

Villar-García, J., J. J. Hernández, R. Güerri-Fernández, A. González, E. Lerma, A. Guelar, D. Saenz, et al. "Effect of probiotics (*Saccharomyces boulardii*) on microbial translocation and inflammation in HIV-treated patients: A double-blind, randomized, placebo-controlled trial." *Journal of Acquired Immune Deficiency Syndromes* 68, no. 3 (2015): 256–63.

Wright S., J. Maree, and M. Sibanyoni. "Treatment of oral thrush in HIV/AIDS patients with lemon juice and lemon grass (*Cymbopogon citratus*) and gentian violet." *Phytomedicine* 16, nos. 2–3 (2009): 118–24.

CHAPTER 6

The Anticandida Diet

Before examining dietary strategies related to candida problems, it is important to comment on the need for a sound
environment for digestion in the stomach. Many people who
suffer from indigestion and heartburn are not in fact the vic-
tims of excessive acid but of too little, and their symptoms represent what happens when (1) food is not adequately digested
in the stomach, leading to excessive fermentation and gas, and
(2) yeasts are active in an environment that is not sufficiently
acidic to inhibit them.

ASSESSING pH LEVELS

Researchers have showed that *Candida albicans* needs a slightly
alkaline environment to thrive (pH of 7.4), while in a strongly
acid environment (pH of 4.5) it is completely inactivated.
People taking antacid medication may therefore be encouraging yeast activity in their stomachs and digestive tracts.

Doctors Stephen Davies and Alan Stewart, in their book
*Nutritional Medicine: The Drug-Free Guide to Better Family
Health,* list some of the common conditions associated with
too little hydrochloric acid. These include asthma, food allergies, iron and vitamin B_{12} deficiency (and therefore fatigue),
bacterial and yeast bowel overgrowth, arthritic symptoms,

diabetes, underactive thyroid gland, bowel sensitivity, and eczema. Among the causes of inadequate acid secretion in the stomach can be exposure to toxic pollution (such as DDT), marijuana smoking, and excessive coffee consumption.

Inadequate stomach acid or an allergic condition can show up as bloating and acid-stomach symptoms. As a first step in normalizing such a problem, the strategy is to take hydrochloric acid (betaine HCL) capsules with each meal. If this eases symptoms significantly, then an herbal method for stimulating the production of digestive acid is suggested, which involves taking a teaspoonful of Swedish bitters (a combination of bitter herbs such as dandelion) two or three times daily, about twenty minutes before eating.

Digestive Enzymes

A second, supplemental digestive strategy may also be useful, especially if food intolerances or allergies are present. This calls for taking natural enzymes—chemicals that we produce to break down foods—which may be inadequately available for a variety of reasons. A broad-spectrum enzyme combination (available from health-food stores and pharmacies) is suggested for anyone with food sensitivities or allergy symptoms.

TWO DIETARY APPROACHES

There are two primary dietary approaches that must be considered in treating candida overgrowth. The first, and most important, involves controlling dietary sugar intake. This approach applies to anyone with a candida problem, without exception, and is among the most important ways to reduce its activity.

The second strategy is appropriate if there is the possibility that you may have become sensitized or allergic to yeast and its byproducts because of your candida overgrowth. This is more likely if your condition is chronic and ongoing, and if the mucous membranes of your intestinal tract have become irritated or even damaged by the invasive fungal form of candida. If this is the case, then avoid foods derived from yeast or contaminated with mold for a period of months.

Both doctors Truss and Crook strongly advocate the dietary approach to treatment of candida, especially to prevent it from spreading. They are also supportive of desensitization methods. My own view is that the dietary approach alone, as set out here, combined with the anticandida methods described in the previous chapter, offer the most effective and safest way forward for anyone with a health problem caused by aggressive yeast overgrowth.

FOODS DERIVED FROM OR CONTAINING FUNGI AND YEAST

Foods and substances that contain yeast or yeastlike substances should be avoided as much as possible, particularly during the initial stages of dealing with candida, and if you know you are sensitive to them. It is probably wise to maintain vigilance about these foods for at least three months, after which time a degree of relaxation can be exercised, with the proviso that if such foods are reintroduced and the symptoms that had lessened begin to manifest again, you should return to a stricter mode of eating for a longer period of time.

The rationale behind avoiding these foods is that they seem to aggravate a candida-induced condition, especially if allergic symptoms are part of the picture, as well as if there are symptoms such as bloating and intestinal gas. In a personal communication Dr. Truss told me, "If someone has no symptoms, I see no reason to have him avoid these yeast-promoting foods, although I will say that in excess, and combined with a high-carbohydrate intake [sugars, etc.], these may actually induce this condition [candida infection] even without the stimulatory effects of antibiotics, birth-control pills, cortisone, etc."

YEAST-PROMOTING FOODS AND SUBSTANCES

The following foods may contain yeast in their preparations and are therefore undesirable, especially in the early stages of an anticandida program:

- Aged meats (sausage, bacon, etc.)
- Any baked good with baker's yeast (pizza dough, bread, etc., including most sourdough breads)
- Anything fermented (vinegar, alcohol, bean paste, soy sauce, etc.)
- B vitamins, unless stated that they are not from yeast
- Barley malt
- Beer
- Black tea
- Blackberries (because of sugar content, see page 126)
- Blueberries (because of sugar content, see page 126)
- Buttermilk
- Canned or bottled juices
- Cheese (all kinds)
- Cider

- Citric acid (this used to be made from citrus juice, but is now made from fermented corn)
- Dried fruits such as apricots, figs, or raisins
- Flavor enhancer (usually MSG, though it may also be yeast extract)
- Ginger ale
- Grapes (because of sugar content, see page 126)
- Jams/jellies
- Lactic acid (generally made from fermented corn or potatoes)
- Liquor
- Malt
- Malted barley flour
- MSG (produced from fermentation of starch or sugar)
- Mushrooms
- Olives
- Peanuts and peanut products
- Preserved or pickled foods
- Raisins
- Root beer
- Soy sauce, miso, tamari
- Strawberries (because of sugar content, see page 126)
- Tempeh
- Vinegar (and foods containing vinegar, such as olives, mustard, ketchup, etc.)
- Wine
- Yeast extract (autolyzed, hydrolyzed)
- Yeast spreads such as Vegemite or Marmite

Note: There is some disagreement among experts as to the wisdom of excluding vinegar and similar products, because there is evidence that a variety of pickled and fermented, plant-based products have probiotic influences, including kombucha (fermented) tea, sauerkraut, miso soup, pickled ginger, cucumbers, and cabbage. And there are certainly benefits to be gained by taking apple cider vinegar—but only if no negative reactions are observed. A simple test would be to introduce it (a teaspoon in warm water two or three times daily) and to note any changes in your symptoms.

The following are either derived from yeast or contain elements that are derived from it, and so should be avoided for at least three months of the anticandida regime if you show any sign of a sensitivity to yeasts or molds:

- Some antibiotics
- Multivitamin tablets (unless specifically stating that they are from a nonyeast source)
- B-complex vitamins
- Individual B-vitamins
- Selenium

Dr. Truss singles out some foods from this long list as the main culprits. He told me, "It is my belief that there are several foods that are primarily to be avoided. These include all fermented drinks, as well as vinegar, mushrooms, and moldy cheeses. I allow my patients to have cottage cheese, as well as yogurt. It is rational to remove all of these foods from the diet only if there is an indication that patients are having trouble with yeast candida."

Finally, nuts, other than freshly cracked ones, should also be avoided, because of the degree of mold that these attract as they become rancid. For that matter, any foods that have been sitting around for a while, other than in a frozen state, are liable to be slightly moldy, and these should be avoided too.

ELIMINATION/CHALLENGE/ROTATION

If you have any doubts about whether any of these foods are likely to be a problem for you, there are two ways of testing this:

1. You should eliminate that food for at least one week and then reintroduce it twice in one day. If no reaction occurs (for example, palpitations, sudden fatigue, brain fog, or the return over the next twenty-four hours of symptoms that have been absent or quiescent), then you can probably include the food in your diet once again. The safest way to do this would be in a rotation pattern, in which you eat the food no more than once in four or five days, until the program is well established—say after three months.

2. You should eliminate the food (or the entire food family, such as dairy, grains, or yeasts) for a week, then reintroduce the foods into your normal diet for several weeks. Once again, you must monitor your symptoms (see chapter 7 for details on how to record symptom scores). If you felt better (i.e., had reduced symptom scores) after a week of avoidance of the food(s) and started to develop the symptoms again after a few days of eating it/them, this is confirmation that the food(s) should be eliminated for several months before attempting them again.

SUGAR-RICH FOODS

Until about a hundred years ago, the average annual intake of sugar in Western countries was in the region of twenty pounds per person. And this was only a part of a dietary pattern that included far more natural, fresh, vitamin- and mineral-rich foods than is currently the case. The present annual intake of sugar in the United States is over a hundred pounds per person! The human body is a marvel of adaptability, but it takes more than a century to get used to such a radical change.

Sugar (sucrose), in whatever guise, is to be strictly avoided during the battle to control candida. This means white sugar, brown sugar, black sugar, and any shades in between. There is no such thing as a healthy sugar. We do not need sugar, as such, for health, and its sole claim for our attention is its taste, which it is quite easy to do without. All sugars aid the growth and proliferation of yeast. This also includes syrups, honey (yes, I'm afraid so), and other forms of sugar such as fructose, maltose, glucose, sorbitol, etc. It includes molasses, date sugar, maple sugar, and in fact all of that range of nonfoods with which our real foods and beverages have been sweetened. Sweets, chocolates, and all soft drinks should obviously be totally avoided. For those unable to tame their desire for sweeteners, there is the option of using stevia, which has nutritional value while not encouraging yeast proliferation.

The undesirability of eating yeast-containing foods removes from the scene bread, pastry, biscuits, cakes, and other baked goods. This is doubly necessary since these are in the main undesirable because of their high carbohydrate content (unless totally whole grain). Basically, any carbohydrate that has been refined beyond the simple grinding stage is undesirable. The more of these foods there are in the diet, the greater the chances of spreading candida.

On the other hand, whole wheat, oats (as employed in making porridge), millet, and brown rice are all highly desirable foods, rich in what are known as complex carbohydrates. These can, and indeed should (especially oats), be a part of the diet. Breads made with sprouted whole grains, such as Ezekiel bread, can be a healthy addition to the diet as well. Note, however, that once these desirable grains are broken down into fine flours and are refined further, they become much less desirable and actually become food for the yeast, rather than for you.

So even in the middle stages of the program when, hopefully, your symptoms are on the wane and you might justifiably feel that you can relax the stricter aspects of your diet somewhat, please remember that refined carbohydrates are the natural food of yeast, and candida will thank you for delivering its favorite foods with a return to heightened activity.

Many foods have "hidden" sugar, in that there is sugar added in the processing or preparation of the food. These are often foods with which sugar is not usually associated. Frozen peas, most canned foods, and many packaged and processed foods all contain either refined flour products or sugar, or both. For this reason, as well as for the general undesirability of many such foods from a nutritional viewpoint, these should be avoided. Not only are you actually providing the favorite foods of the yeasts within your body when you eat sugar, you are also causing a degree of metabolic and physiological mayhem.

The pancreas, the source of insulin and essential

protein-digesting enzymes, becomes grossly overworked when sugar plays a large part in the diet. When faced with sugar, the pancreas pumps out insulin, which maintains the proper level of sugar in the bloodstream. Insulin is also released in response to stimulant drinks such as coffee and tea, which initially cause a release by the liver of stored sugar (as does stress). Thus a diet rich in sugar, which also contains the usual pattern of tea, coffee, and alcohol (as well as cola drinks and chocolates, which also contain caffeine), will produce a situation in which a major organ is grossly overworked. In this scenario the fluctuations in blood sugar levels, boosted by dietary sugar and the sugar stored in the liver, and then depressed and controlled by the pancreatic insulin, have a profound effect on a person's health and personality. At the same time it is noted that a sugar-rich diet makes it much less likely that a person will eat enough foods containing vitamins and minerals to allow him or her to meet the minimum standards of nutrition. Thus other systems in the body become deficient, including the immune system. This whole process may, of course, take years, all the while accompanied by declining well-being and an unseen rise in candida activity. No wonder sugar has been described as "pure, white, and deadly."

What about Fruit?

It is suggested that in the first few weeks of the program (say the first three weeks) even fresh fruit should be avoided because of its high content of natural fruit sugars. Even when fruit is resumed after the three-week break, it should exclude the very sweet fruits like melons and grapes, which are too high in sugar for the candida sufferer (and often contain mold).

And Milk Products?

Milk contains its own form of sugar, and this too is thought to be undesirable throughout the program. Pasteurized milk encourages candida. The exception to this is yogurt, as long as it is natural and live, which will be clearly stated on its container. Live yogurt inhibits candida and assists in the repopulation of the bowel flora. There are many "dead" yogurts around, and a good many that have added sugar as well as sugar-containing fruits. These are quite unsuitable to the program.

A Low-Sugar Diet Helps to Control Yeast

In one study published in the *Journal of Reproductive Medicine,* it was found that of a hundred women with candida-induced vaginitis the levels of glucose and other sugar breakdown products excreted correlated with the amount of dairy products, artificial sweeteners, and sugars the women consumed. When they were placed on a diet that eliminated these there were "dramatic reductions in the incidence and severity of their illness."

While it is well known that diabetics are prone to yeast infections in general, and candida in particular, it has also been shown that nondiabetics whose blood sugar is on the high side of normal are also prone to yeast infections. Quite simply, although they are not considered diabetic, many people have poor glucose tolerance, and yeast therefore proliferates.

As mentioned in chapter 5, chromium supplementation (glucose tolerance factor, 200 mcg daily), as well as avoiding sugary foods, should help to keep blood sugar balanced and candida under control.

AN ANTICANDIDA DIET PLAN

With a little creativity and motivation, you can eat foods that are varied and exciting as part of your anticandida program. Below I have outlined an anticandida diet that is tasty and nutritious. Once you have followed this diet for a while it is quite possible that you will never want to reintroduce the old "undesirables" again, even when candida is back under control, because you will feel so much better without eating those foods.

Try to eat three meals a day, and don't skip a meal unless you are ill or have no appetite.

Breakfast

A high-fiber diet is best suited to the resolution of any candida problem. Choose therefore from one or more of the following for a wholesome breakfast that does not encourage candida proliferation:

Oatmeal: Make with water, not milk. Add a little cinnamon and some fresh ground nuts for additional flavor. Use no sugar or honey. Add several spoonfuls of fructooligosaccharides (FOS), which have a slightly sweet taste, to feed your friendly bacteria. Stevia may also be safely added, in liquid or powder form.

Mixed seed and nut breakfast: Combine sunflower, pumpkin, sesame, and flax seeds together with oatmeal or flaked millet. These can be eaten as they are or soaked overnight in a little water to make a softer texture, or moistened with natural live yogurt. Add wheat germ and freshly milled nuts, and FOS or stevia, if desired.

Eggs: On alternate days, two eggs, any style except raw

Bread/toast: Bread made without yeast or sugar (including sprouted whole grain breads like Ezekiel), and butter

Brown rice kedgeree: A rice and fish dish

Whole wheat or rice and oat pancakes (no sweet toppings)

Natural live yogurt or fromage fraiche: Add a dessert-spoonful of coldpressed flaxseed oil, blend well, and then add flax and other seeds. This makes an energy-rich power breakfast and is highly recommended (as long as you have no sensitivity to dairy products).

Fresh fruit: After the first three weeks or so of the program fresh fruit can be added to the menu. For example, to an oatmeal or a mixed seed-and-nut breakfast you could add sliced banana or grated apple; fresh fruit could be added to live yogurt; or fruit could be eaten as a major part of the meal, with a handful of fresh nuts and/or seeds (sunflower, pumpkin, etc.). Continue to avoid fruit juices, however.

Fish and meat: No smoked, cured, or salted meats or conventional "factory-farmed" animal products (more on this in the next section).

Whole wheat or whole rice flakes and yogurt: Muesli-type breakfast cereals are in order, but only if they are homemade. If store-bought they will most likely contain dried fruit (sugar) and nuts of almost certain rancidity, and frequently added sugar or honey. By simply mixing oat or millet flakes with fresh nuts or seeds, as mentioned above, it is possible to have a high-fiber, nutritious, tasty meal. If you're eating an oatmeal or a mixed seed-and-nut breakfast, then you are eating high-fiber foods, which are the most desirable. If any of the other choices are eaten, then add a heaping teaspoonful of half flax seeds and half bran mixed together and added to the cereal, or eat separately at the end of the meal with a little water.

Remember to chew all food thoroughly, especially carbohydrates. There is no way that half-chewed carbohydrates can be digested, since the enzymes present in saliva are essential for the breakdown of these foods. For this reason it is undesirable to drink with meals, as the liquid is frequently used as a moistening agent to facilitate swallowing, which reduces efficient chewing.

A high-fiber meal is ideal for an anticandida program. It provides a steady release of natural sugars into the bloodstream, rather than the rapid rise produced by most refined sugar-rich foods. This helps to keep blood-sugar levels even, and avoids ups and downs in available energy (and mood), which can be a major cause of the craving for a quick sugar fix.

Beverages at breakfast time should consist of either green tea, pau d'arco tea, china tea, herb tea (such as rooibos or chamomile)—all unsweetened—or mineral water. Avoid fruit juices unless diluted 50:50 with water, and even then not for the first two weeks of the program. In addition to these kinds of liquids, drink no less than 1.5 and ideally up to 2.5 quarts (liters) of spring or filtered water daily, mainly between meals.

Main Meals: Lunch and Dinner

There should be no obstacles to eating delicious, nutritious food even during the strict avoidance period of the dietary program.

Animal proteins: One area of contention exists in the choice of animal proteins. It is important to realize that most commercial meat, poultry, pork, and eggs contain residues of antibiotics and hormonal substances, which are fed to the animals in the process of rearing them for market. This means that unless you eat organic, grass-fed, or pasture-raised animal products, and organic, hormone-free dairy products, you are endangering the success of your whole program, not to mention adding health hazards. Indeed, it is not improbable that this very factor is a major, if as yet under-recognized, element in the whole candida scenario. While the use of antibiotics and steroids in medications can be relatively easily traced in one's medical history, it is impossible to know just how much of these same substances people are consuming on a daily basis in the food they eat.

For this reason it is important that you eat only organic, grass-fed meats, poultry, and dairy products and nonfarmed fish (farmed fish contain antibiotics). Today most cities and even smaller towns have grocery stores that provide healthy options, including meat and poultry free of all contamination. Note that lamb and mutton is less likely to have added hormones, and wild meat such as rabbit and other game meats or poultry are usually quite acceptable and often preferable. Wild-caught fish is also safe (if it hasn't been exposed to other environmental toxins). For the duration of the diet, therefore, it is suggested that unless the source of fish, meat, or poultry can be identified with certainty as being free of hormones or antibiotics, all meat consumption should be limited to wild game, mutton or lamb, and wild-caught fish.

Vegetables: Ideally, in order to maintain the high-fiber type of meal that is so desirable when candida is active, the two main meals of the day should include as wide a variety of fresh vegetables as is possible. These should be eaten both raw and cooked, and an excellent pattern to adopt is as follows. One of the main meals (say lunch) can be a source of protein such as fish, poultry, lamb, eggs, or fresh nuts, together with as large a mixed salad as your imagination can conjure up and your appetite can handle. The other main meal should also include protein, in addition to cooked vegetables. The source of protein at each meal does not of course have to be based on animals. The combining of a cereal and a pulse (say brown rice and lentils, or millet and chickpeas) at the same meal ensures that adequate protein is available to the body. Note that pulses are part of the legume family, but the term *pulse* refers only to the dried seed. Dried peas, edible beans, lentils, and chickpeas are the most common varieties of pulses. Pulses are very high in protein and fiber and are low in fat.

What is essential, though, is that adequate protein is eaten daily, whether from a safe animal source or from the careful mixing of complementary vegetable proteins. Note that what is adequate for one person is not necessarily so for another. For example, people of Asian ancestry require, for good health, less protein than people of Northern European stock. The difference lies in the efficiency with which people digest and absorb what proteins they eat. Thus 50 g a day of first-class protein is adequate for an East Asian person, while 75 g (or more depending on activity, etc.) may be required by someone of Northern European ancestry.

Since natural live yogurt (a source of protein and probiotics) is going to play an important part of the diet, eating protein at both of the main meals, in addition to eating yogurt, is not necessary. It should be possible to have, for example, a mixed salad, together with a jacket potato or savory rice dish, and additional nuts and seeds for one meal, while having an animal protein and a variety of cooked vegetables for the other main meal. In any case, the tastes and preferences of individual people will differ markedly, and the variations that are possible as to what to eat are so great that no more than broad guidelines can be given.

The essential guidelines for your main meals are as follows:

- Avoid all yeast-based or yeast-containing foods (unless certain that there is no sensitivity to these).
- Avoid all sugar and refined cereal products, and foods containing them.
- Avoid all foods and drinks based on fermentation (with the exception of cider vinegar and the pickled/fermented foods such as sauerkraut).
- Avoid absolutely all meat, poultry, and fish that contains residues of antibiotics and steroids.
- Eat three meals daily.
- Ensure adequate protein intake.
- Ensure that a high dietary fiber content is maintained.
- Avoid fruit for the first three or four weeks of the program.

Increasing the Variety of Foods

Once symptoms of candida overgrowth begin to subside, usually after two months or so, and you find that you would like to increase the range of foods slightly, it is of course permissible to experiment a bit. However, this should not be done before the end of the second month on the program, and it should only be done if there has been a marked improvement in your condition. If you then introduce one food that has been on the "no" list, observe the consequences carefully. If these are nonexistent, you might extend your experiment to another food after a week or so. If symptoms return, go back to basic avoidance until the symptoms calm down again. I am not saying that you *must* experiment in this way, only that if you feel constrained by the limitations imposed by the diet, then at least introduce such foods carefully, with the knowledge that they might interfere with your progress. If they do, this just means you must be patient and persevere in the program.

There are many excellent books available that explain the principles of rotation diets, which can help you to formulate a strategy for eating certain foods only periodically, in a systematic way. It is not suggested that the reintroduction of sugar-containing foods be started at this stage, other than in the very minimal sense—or perhaps introducing only a little honey.

Other Essential Information Regarding Food

Mold is present on most fruits and vegetables, and therefore these should be kept well washed and eaten fresh, for the longer they are stored, the more likely it is that mold will develop. Nuts are also subject to mold (in the case of peanuts this is a highly toxic, potentially cancer-causing agent). All nuts, unless freshly opened by you, will contain some degree of mold, and certainly a degree of rancidity of the natural oils. Eat current-season nuts, freshly opened by yourself, or nuts and seeds such as pumpkin, sunflower, and so forth, that have been kept continuously refrigerated, or else avoid them entirely.

As well, yeasts and mold also grow on grains of all sorts, and so the fresher the grains the better. A good many people with candida problems are allergic to grains. This allergy may well diminish during the program of candida control, and a little experimentation is in order after two or three months if your symptoms generally have declined.

Apart from a little butter and natural live yogurt, it is suggested that all milk products be avoided (although some experts allow cottage cheese).

If you happen to go to a restaurant, or if friends invite you over for a meal, make sure you stick to the basics. Avoid sauces and gravy; avoid desserts; avoid things like stuffing (as in turkey stuffing), or any obvious undesirables, such as mushrooms. A meat, poultry, or fish dish, with salad or vegetables, is the safest bet, and stick to water instead of wine.

What about sugar substitutes for those with a sweet tooth? Fructooligosaccharides (FOS) are sweet and do not encourage yeast. FOS can safely be added to foods for sweetness, as can stevia.

Remember that all commercial breakfast foods (corn flakes, etc.) are undesirable. They are processed, and most contain yeast and/or sugar products.

Water from the tap should be filtered before drinking if possible. There are many inexpensive water filters available that will remove a variety of organic substances that otherwise find their way into food, or directly into you. Most bottled water is acceptable, but make sure this is not carbonated if you have problems with bloating and gas. As for coffee and tea, this is a sticking point for many people. Both are undesirable, not only as sources of mold (in the case of tea), but because they stimulate sugar release from the liver.

Herbal teas are often better, and some have been found to help in the control of candida and related problems, such as rooibos, a South African tea, and pau d'arco, which is helpful in catarrhal problems caused by candida. Additionally there are a number of healthy coffee "substitutes" (herbal roasts) available in good health-food stores, such as Ayurvedic Roast (ayurvedicroast.com).

Steaming vegetables is the best way to retain their vital minerals so often destroyed and lost in boiling. Dressing a salad with lemon juice, olive oil, and a little natural yogurt can replace the vinegar or other dressings not compatible with the program.

As the program produces its results, and symptoms become tolerable, or disappear, so can a limited quantity of foods based on or containing mold or yeast be reintroduced. Wine, or real ale, in limited amounts, or tea, etc., may be taken occasionally. However, the need for vigilance must continue, because it is not the aim of the program to remove candida from the scene altogether, nor would this even be possible, as there is always a certain amount of this yeast in the body even under normal conditions.

The long-term solution, after initially controlling the yeast overgrowth by the methods outlined in this book, is to maintain a high level of immune function through your diet, in terms of its nutrient value, as well as to avoid those factors that you now know can reduce its optimum functioning of the immune system. This does not mean that the anticandida program is a life sentence. It is hoped that after a while your palette will change and you will come to regard sweet tastes as unsatisfying, no longer craving or even enjoying sweet foods like you used to. It is also hoped that your newfound sense of well-being will help motivate you to more or less follow the diet suggested here on a permanent basis, not only because it is good for you, but because you have actually come to enjoy it.

Environmental Factors

It is important not only to avoid foods and drinks that contain fungal or yeast substances but also to avoid inhaling these organisms. For this reason keep well away from damp, dank places and don't personally deal with mold or wet or dry rot if it is present in your environment (many towns and cities offer mold removal services). If there is any danger of dampness in rooms, cupboards, cellars, or lofts, eliminate this, or, if necessary, move to a new, dry place of residence. Please consider that your home might be making you ill. This advice is especially applicable to anyone whose symptoms get worse in damp or muggy weather, or who is obviously affected by contact with moldy or dank environments.

Exercise

The immune system benefits when you get adequate exercise. At least every other day there should be a form of physical exercise sufficient to stimulate the circulation and respiration. A brisk walk for ten minutes or more is the safest and easiest form of exercise that can produce such immune-system benefits, while cycling, swimming, yoga, tai chi, Pilates, etc., all offer a chance to move and use the body beneficially.

Stress

Avoiding or managing stress and anxiety is fundamental for a healthy life, a widely documented fact. For this reason any and all methods that encourage relaxation, such as meditation, yoga, tai chi, a good long walk in a park, etc., are recommended.

Motivation

The degree to which someone can adhere to an anticandida diet depends on many factors, but none less than motivation. Just how much do you want to get better, and just how much effort are you prepared to make in this quest? It is really not up to anyone but you. Certainly by taking supplements, as described, you will go a long way toward that end. Avoiding yeasts and foods derived from them will also help greatly. But by putting the whole program together, including the sugar-free aspect of the diet, you really give the whole process a chance to work quickly, and well.

LITERATURE

Beer, M. F., F. M. Frank, O. Germán Elso, et al. "Trypanocidal and leishmanicidal activities of flavonoids isolated from *Stevia satureiifolia* var. satureiifolia." *Pharmaceutical Biology* 17 (2016): 1–8.

Berkhof, I., M. van Dusseldorp, C. M. Swanink, and J. W. van der Meer. "A diet for chronic fatigue caused by *Candida albicans?*" *Nederlands Tijdschrift voor Geneeskunde* 135, no. 43 (1991): 2017–19.

Bland, Jeffrey, ed. *Medical Applications of Clinical Nutrition*. New Canaan, Conn.: Keats, 1983.

Bodey, Gerald P., ed. "Candidiasis in the Gastrointestinal Tract." In *Candidiasis: Pathogenesis, Diagnosis, and Treatment*. New York: Raven Press, 1992.

Davies, Stephen, and Alan Stewart. *Nutritional Medicine: The Drug-Free Guide to Better Family Health*. London: Pan Books, 1987.

Chen, Wei Chung, and Eamonn M. M. Quigley. "Probiotics, prebiotics and synbiotics in small intestinal bacterial overgrowth:

Opening up a new therapeutic horizon!" *Indian Journal of Medical Research* 140, no. 5 (2014): 582.

Crook, William. *The Yeast Connection: A Medical Breakthrough.* New York: Vintage, 1986.

———, Carolyn Dean, and Elizabeth Crook. *The Yeast Connection and Women's Health.* New York: Square One, 2007.

Hobday, R. A., S. Thomas, A. O'Donovan, M. Murphy, and A. J. Pinching. "Dietary intervention in chronic fatigue syndrome." *Journal of Human Nutrition and Dietetics* 21, no. 2 (2008): 141–49.

Horowitz, B., S. W. Edelstein, and L. Lippman. "Sugar chromatography studies in recurrent *Candida* vulvovaginitis." *Journal of Reproductive Medicine* 29, no. 7 (1984): 441–43.

Kadir, T., R. Pisiriciler, S. Akyüz, A. Yarat, N. Emekli, and A. Ipbüker. "Mycological and cytological examination of oral candidal carriage in diabetic patients and non-diabetic control subjects: Thorough analysis of local aetiologic and systemic factors." *Journal of Oral Rehabilitation* 29, no. 5 (2002): 452–57.

Katahn, Martin. *The Rotation Diet.* New York: W. W. Norton, 2012.

Lefèvre, L., A. Galès, D. Olagnier, J. Bernad, L. Perez, R. Burcelin, A. Valentin, J. Auwerx, B. Pipy, and A. Coste. "PPARγ ligands switched high fat diet-induced macrophage M2b polarization toward M2a thereby improving intestinal *Candida* elimination." *PLoS One* 5, no. 9 (2010): e12828.

Macura, A. B., T. Gasińska, B. Pawlik, and A. Obłoza. "Nail susceptibility to fungal infection in patients with type 1 and 2 diabetes under long term poor glycaemia control." *Przeglad Lekarski* 64, no. 6 (2007): 406–9.

Martins de Lima-Salgado, T., S. Coccuzzo Sampaio, M. F. Cury-Boaventura, and R. Curi. "Modulatory effect of fatty acids on fungicidal activity, respiratory burst and TNF-α and IL-6 production in J774 murine macrophages." *British Journal of Nutrition* 105, no. 8 (2011): 1173–79.

Petitpierre, M., P. Gumowski, and J. P. Girard. "Irritable bowel syndrome and hypersensitivity to food." *Annals of Allergy* 54, no. 6 (1985): 538–40.

Ritu, M., and J. Nandini. "Nutritional composition of *Stevia rebaudiana,* a sweet herb and its hypoglycaemic and hypolipidaemic effect on patients with non insulin dependent diabetes mellitus." *Journal of the Science of Food and Agriculture* (2016). doi: 10.1002/jsfa.7627.

Truss, C. Orion. *The Missing Diagnosis II.* C. Orion Truss, 2009.

Villena, J., S. Salva, G. Agüero, and S. Alvarez. "Immunomodulatory and protective effect of probiotic *Lactobacillus casei* against *Candida albicans* infection in malnourished mice." *Microbiology and Immunology* 55, no. 6 (2011): 434–45.

Weig, M., E. Werner, M. Frosch, and H. Kasper. "Limited effect of refined carbohydrate dietary supplementation on colonization of the gastrointestinal tract of healthy subjects by *Candida albicans.*" *American Journal of Clinical Nutrition* 69, no. 6 (1999): 1170–73.

Yamaguchi, N., K. Sonoyama, H. Kikuchi, T. Nagura, T. Aritsuka, and J. Kawabata. "Gastric colonization of *Candida albicans* differs in mice fed commercial and purified diets." *Journal of Nutrition* 135, no. 1 (2005): 109–15.

CHAPTER 7

Putting Your Total Anticandida Program Together

❦

A Ten-Point Plan

To get a strong indication as to whether *Candida albicans* overgrowth is a factor in your health problems, carefully answer the questionnaire in chapter 4. The following suggestions do not take into account every possible variation but can be used as a guide as to what is likely to be successful in controlling candida in most instances.

The strongest recommendation I can make is that you consult an expert in the treatment of yeast and fungal problems. Try to find someone to consult with who is either a naturopathic practitioner with sound qualifications, a nutritionally trained medical practitioner (such as a clinical ecologist), a homeopath who employs nutritional methods, a well-qualified nutritionist, or some other health care professional with appropriate knowledge and experience. And if you're considering consulting with someone, don't hesitate to ask for details about the person's qualifications and experience.

If money is an issue or you don't have an expert practitioner in your area, you can still self-treat, but I urge you not to take a pick-and-choose approach to an anticandida program; rather, you should comprehensively follow all elements of the anticandida program as outlined in this book. This means incorporating all of the following:

- Antifungal methods
- Detoxification plus liver and immune support
- Repopulation with probiotic organisms
- A basic anticandida diet
- Use of additional local treatment methods as indicated (such as healing the mucous membrane if there is leaky gut syndrome)

KEEPING TRACK OF SYMPTOMS

List your major symptoms on the left-hand side of a sheet of paper; underline each one and extend that line clear across the page. Then draw columns (vertical lines down the page) that divide the page up into a series of boxes into which, each day, next to each symptom, you can enter a score regarding its intensity over the past twenty-four hours. At the top of each of these columns enter the date on which you are scoring your symptoms, and next to the symptom enter a value—for example, you might decide that the worst your thrush irritation can ever be is equal to a score of 3, and that when there are no symptoms at all you would score a 0. Then you can decide for yourself what score you would give to a symptom.

Be sure to enter all your symptoms on the left side of the page—for example, indigestion, fatigue, headache, muscle pain, and so on.

Leave the very bottom of the page, the last inch or so, open, and in that space, under the appropriate date, you can enter both a total symptom score (add up all your individual scores for that day) as well as any short notes or reminders, such as "started acidophilus," "my period started," "got a cold," "ran out of caprylic acid," or anything else that will jog your memory when you look back at your scores weeks or months later, so you can see what factors influenced your scores. I suggest that you keep this scoresheet handy and fill it in at the same time each day, say just before your evening meal or at bedtime.

SAMPLE SYMPTOM SCORESHEET

SYMPTOM	DATE	DATE	DATE	DATE	DATE	DATE	DATE	DATE	DATE	DATE
Tired	3	3	3	2	2	1	2	1	2	1
Gas	3	3	3	2	2	2	0	1	2	1
Head	1	1	2	1	3	2	3	1	1	1
Runs	1	1	3	3	1	0	1	0	2	0
Skin-itch	1	0	0	0	3	0	1	1	1	0
PMS	3	3	3	2	2	1	1	0	1	0
Sore mouth	2	2	2	2	1	1	1	2	1	0
Other	?	?	?	?	?	?	?	?	?	?
Other	?	?	?	?	?	?	?	?	?	?
Total	14	13	16	12	14	7	9	6	10	3
Notes	started program				period began					

This sample table gives you an idea of how you can keep track of your symptoms and the individual aspects of your program as they affect your health.

The value of this method of symptom scoring is enormous, since as you make changes in your program you can judge their impact on your individual symptoms as well as on your total score. This helps to unravel the sometimes complicated causative elements. For example, you may have five or six symptoms listed, and only three of these may have changed markedly within the first few months of the program. This tells you that the symptoms that improved probably relate directly to your candida overgrowth, while the others do not, and therefore require some other form of attention.

It is also useful to remind yourself where you have been in terms of the intensity of symptoms as the weeks pass by. A satisfactory slow decline of scores is very gratifying (with minor ups and downs, which can occur for many reasons). It is also important to know if scores do not decline, since this may be a sign that either the problem is not candida-related, or that the program you are undertaking is inadequate. In either case it is better to realize this sooner rather than later.

If your condition is severe, don't expect major beneficial changes before two months on the program; in fact, your scores could even increase for the first few weeks during the initial stages of candida elimination, as die-off occurs and the detoxification process begins. This is known as Herxheimer's reaction, and it may include general flulike symptoms such as malaise, nausea, aching limbs, depression, or an apparent flare-up of previous symptoms in areas where candida had colonized. This happens when infecting agents are killed and the toxins are released faster than the kidneys and liver can remove them via the natural detoxification process. Such a reaction soon after starting an anticandida program (i.e., within a few days) should be considered a normal side effect and is an indication of a likely positive outcome if you stick with it.

Take It in Stages

Since the comprehensive antifungal program presented here calls for a great many changes, and since all of them are potentially stressful to some extent, as your body gets accustomed to the changes it is best to introduce elements of the program in stages, first eliminating allergens, then reducing and cutting out sugars, then introducing immune-enhancing nutrients, then perhaps after two to three weeks introducing liver-support strategies and the pre- and probiotics, followed by antifungal methods (more on this below).

All of this can take several weeks to get into place, and it is to be expected that some odd symptoms might appear during this time, especially regarding altered bowel function, abdominal noises, and probably some degree of nausea and/or headaches and fatigue in excess of what you have previously noted. These changes indicate the onset of the detoxification process and should not be cause for anxiety—and they certainly should not stop you from proceeding. This is where expert advice and support can be so helpful, especially if you are trying to manage all these changes singlehandedly, without the emotional and practical support that is so useful during such a time.

The beginning is a particularly important phase of the program, when it is tempting to give up. Knowing in advance that symptoms might flare up, and that overall you might feel worse before you feel better, should encourage you to persevere with the plan.

A TEN-POINT STRATEGY

First, reduce or stop using completely (after consulting your medical adviser) any steroid medications or antibiotics.
Then:

1. If you regularly suffer from indigestion, heartburn, acid stomach, or bloating, consider the methods outlined in chapter 6 regarding supplementing with betaine HCL or Swedish bitters to see whether these problems are not in fact due to inadequate acid supply.
2. If you experience allergic/sensitivity symptoms, introduce a broad-spectrum enzyme supplement with each main meal and assess the benefits over a period of several weeks.
3. If you are sensitive to yeast-type foods, eliminate these (per the lists in chapter 6) for at least two and ideally three months before attempting a challenge and possible rotation of the foods back into your diet. If you are aware that you have dairy or wheat allergies, for example, eliminate these foods altogether for the duration of the first three months of the program, before reassessing their impact.
4. Introduce the sugar-elimination aspects of the anticandida diet as outlined in chapter 6.
5. Introduce immune-enhancing supplementation as outlined in chapter 5.
6. After introducing all of the above over a period of four to eight weeks, as appropriate to your condition, all the while assessing symptom scores as discussed at the beginning of this chapter, begin incorporating the other elements of the diet, as follows:

- Introduce probiotic supplementation as outlined in chapter 5.
- Introduce antifungal strategies as outlined in chapter 5.
- If there are symptoms indicating bowel irritation (such as food sensitivities and/or previous diagnosis of irritable bowel syndrome, and/or mucous in the bowel movements, and/or a longstanding and severe degree of yeast involvement), introduce methods to reduce bowel permeability as outlined in chapter 5.
- If there are local manifestations of yeast involvement, introduce appropriate local measures to address conditions in the mouth, vagina, etc., as discussed in chapter 5.

7. If yeast die-off is severe, there are strategies for reducing the toxic load involving the use of herbal and nutritional support (nutrients such as molybdenum and zinc, or the amino acids L-cysteine or L-methionine and/or L-carnitine, for example), as well as herbal liver support such as milk-thistle extract and/or ginger. If necessary, consider seeking professional nutritional advice.

8. Introduce detoxification methods that are not diet-related, such as skin brushing, Epsom-salt baths, various aromatherapy essential oil baths, etc. Also consider relaxation, breath work, yoga, and other stress-reducing, immune-enhancing methods.

9. If bowel dysbiosis (chronic constipation, for example) is causing increased toxicity, colonic irrigation may be useful at this time, as may coffee enemas. These need to be individually prescribed according to need. As for coffee enemas, seek advice on how to administer these from a qualified professional, as it would be unwise for you to experiment with this method on your own.

10. After two months, a further change in the program may be called for, whereby you introduce modified antifungal strategies depending on your progress. Changes in your diet may also be permissible if sensitivities and symptoms are reduced.

If your symptom scores decline steadily (albeit with ups and downs due to individual circumstances), there is every reason to press on. If symptoms are not markedly improved after at least two months of consistent application of the main elements of this program, it is time to reassess your condition and how you are trying to deal with it. Expert advice is probably called for, if you haven't already sought it out.

How Often Should You Consult a Professional?

Seek expert advice once at the start of, and probably at six- to eight-week intervals during, the three- to six-month course of this program. In severe cases the program may need to be maintained for up to a year, with periodic consultations.

If special needs call for more frequent consultations or treatments, this should be established at the very beginning of the course. Nowadays, once the program is underway, where minor fine-tuning of the program is needed, it is possible to get expert advice via e-mail or Skype calls, thus avoiding the need for face-to-face consultations.

Once candida is under control, a maintenance program is usually called for, during which you will maintain a low-sugar, low-fat diet, with wholesome, nutritious, balanced foods forming the major elements of your diet. At this time some relaxation of the restrictions is usually possible, and the intake of supplemental nutrients is usually reduced to just some probiotic supplementation and possibly a daily multivitamin-mineral nutrient support.

Many thousands of people have benefited from following the advice given in this book. It cannot take the place of individually prescribed methods that take into account your unique health profile and needs, but it is a useful starting point if you have found yourself unable to get help from your regular health advisers. Hopefully, as ever more general practitioners (MDs) become aware of the value of this approach, you will find the support you need. Until then, you must take responsibility, take action, and if necessary seek expert advice from a qualified practitioner.

The "Hardiness Factor"

Candida and its associated symptoms can be exhausting and demoralizing. Gathering the resolve to make changes in your diet and habits calls for energy that you may believe you don't have available. The ideas outlined below might assist you in making those necessary changes. Experts have identified characteristics that have been described as the "hardiness" or "resilience" factor, which comprises three main attributes: challenge, control, and commitment. Some people possess these qualities innately, but if they are not already present in you, they can be acquired.

Challenge: When health problems are seen as challenges to be overcome, there is likely to be motivation to address the causes in positive ways, giving a sense of purpose and meaning to life. The opposite is to see health issues as overwhelming forces that crush you, rather than motivate you. By making a conscious effort to view life more optimistically, your expectations and behavior can change, resulting in more positive outcomes than you may have imagined possible.

Control: This is defined as the extent to which you feel a sense that you have the ability to influence your life for the better. The opposite is to have feelings of powerlessness. When you begin to exercise control over any part of your life (changing your diet is a good example), you move toward control and empowerment, even if this is only temporary and partial at the beginning.

Commitment: This involves having a sense of purpose that motivates you to actively attempt to influence your life and surroundings, and to persevere. This contrasts with having no motivation and no commitment. That you are reading this book and that you are trying to improve your health shows that the germ of commitment is active within you. Nurture it as you explore ways to manage and overcome your health issues.

LITERATURE

Chia, Mantak, and William U. Wei. *Cosmic Detox: A Taoist Approach to Internal Cleansing.* Rochester, Vt.: Destiny Books, 2011.

Clampett, Cheri, and Biff Mithoeffer. *The Therapeutic Yoga Kit: Sixteen Postures for Self-Healing through Quiet Yin Awareness.* Rochester, Vt.: Healing Arts Press, 2009.

Vasey, Christopher. *The Water Prescription.* Rochester, Vt.: Healing Arts Press, 2006.

CHAPTER 8

Ten Case Histories

I trained as a naturopath and osteopath in the United Kingdom, qualifying from the British College of Osteopathic Medicine in 1960. After graduating I studied orthomolecular nutrition, as well as acupuncture. And after a few years working at a residential clinic, where I learned a great deal about the practical holistic care of people with chronic ill health, I launched into private practice on the south coast of England.

As with all clinical experience it was my exposure to the varied range of real-life health concerns that polished my earlier theoretical education, and I slowly became aware of unusual trends in the symptoms my patients were presenting with. "New" conditions were appearing, or rather "old" ones were appearing more often!

In particular, by the late 1970s and early 1980s there were more and more (mainly) female patients reporting chronic unexplained fatigue, digestive complaints, and chronic pain.

As time passed, terms such as *chronic fatigue syndrome, candidiasis,* and *fibromyalgia* became more and more commonly written about and understood, and my practice reflected this. In particular the research and writing of Dr. Crook and Dr. Truss (as described in earlier chapters) revolutionized my understanding of why these conditions were reaching epidemic levels—and what could be done to help those affected.

And as the treatment methods that I employed slowly modified to meet these clinical challenges, the methods outlined in this book were refined. The cases reported in this chapter offer a glimpse of that process.

1. KATE, AGE FORTY-TWO

When she arrived for her first consultation, Kate was accompanied by her husband. At the time she looked so washed-out and aged beyond her years that I took him to be her son. Her hair was lank, she was overweight and what I can only describe as "crumpled." Her symptoms included a range of digestive complaints (intermittent diarrhea/constipation, bloating, indigestion, etc.); various PMS symptoms; backache and neck pain; extreme fatigue; skin rashes (especially under the breasts), which had been diagnosed as yeast related; disturbed sleep involving night sweats and extreme restlessness; depression; as well as vaginitis and thrush. These symptoms were of about fifteen years' duration, and had begun after she had started bearing children (three so far). She was receiving antidepressant medication from her doctor (and had been for over a year), who supported her consulting me for her candida problems.

Kate expressed despair at her condition, saying that she felt she was unable to be a "good wife and mother," the role she had chosen for herself. The program I suggested was a strict application of antifungal strategies (low-sugar, low-fat diet, with abundant complex carbohydrates, including vegetables and whole grains), as well as a low-yeast pattern of eating (she had a history of sensitivity to yeast-based foods). I advised local application of aloe vera juice alternating with diluted tea tree oil on the skin infection areas. I specifically prescribed acidophilus and bifidobacteria, along with caprylic acid and garlic capsules three times daily. A range of immune-supporting nutrients were also suggested.

Kate kept a detailed symptom record sheet, and over the next six months her total score and individual symptom scores progressively declined after an initial ten days during which time she told me, "I thought I was dying," so severe were her die-off symptoms (nausea, headaches, lethargy, restlessness, flulike aches). She phoned me during this initial time of die-off, and I suggested that she temporarily increase her intake of probiotics (bifidobacteria helps liver decongestion) and reduce caprylic acid intake until severe die-off symptoms lessened after a few days, at which time the program could be resumed as before.

By the third month, when I again saw her, Kate was significantly better, although there had been a period of about two weeks during the second month when her symptoms flared up again for no obvious reason. At this point she looked years younger and had lost fourteen pounds without any specific effort in that direction; she had also regained some energy.

The program was kept in place, unmodified for a further three months, at which time her symptoms were virtually absent. Her weight loss was now at over twenty-eight pounds. Her vitality was restored, her skin was clear, and her bowel function normal. She asked me about stopping her antidepressant medication and I suggested she talk to her doctor about this. I wrote to him indicating that I believed that her depression was the result rather than the cause of her condition, and that she could probably be weaned off the drugs altogether if he agreed. When I saw her for the fourth and last time at the end of the ninth month she had a symptom score sheet ranging between one and zero (at the start it had been in the high twenties, relating to eleven symptoms). The one that she was still scoring was because of a periodically furred tongue. Her weight had dropped a total of forty-two pounds, and she had successfully been taken off her antidepressant medication. Her husband (who now looked older than her) was delighted, as were their children, and she informed me they had told her that they were glad to have their mom "back again."

It was at this time that we relaxed her dietary pattern to allow a few treats of the sugary kind, and at her last communication to me she reported that all remained well.

Kate's case illustrates the multisymptomatic pattern that many candida sufferers endure; the possibility that antidepressants are prescribed for what is a symptom and not a cause; and the way in which a dedicated person can put her life back together in the face of enormous health challenges.

Reflecting on Kate's story made me realize that when she first came to me as a patient, the condition we now know as Fibromyalgia Syndrome (FMS) had not been "officially" defined by the medical profession. And yet, if Kate had seen a rheumatologist a few years later it is likely that FMS would have been diagnosed.

Over the past twenty-five years I have seen many patients with such a diagnosis (or with a "chronic fatigue" label) where widespread pain, fatigue, digestive troubles and other symptoms were all present, and where candida was a major feature of their problem—just as it was for Kate.

2. FRANK, AGE THIRTY-FOUR

This young gay man who had been HIV positive for some five years arrived to see me with a single complaint—candida overgrowth in his mouth (thrush) so severe that his tongue and cheeks were covered in white patches. It is well known that with immunosuppression comes yeast activity, and that a manifestation of oral thrush of this sort is quite common among HIV-positive persons and others with different immune-related illnesses. His diet had once been very sugar-oriented, but at the time he saw me he had for the past few months been following a sound health-enhancing diet. He was, however, skipping meals from time to time due to work pressure, and on such days his energy levels were dramatically depleted.

Frank was troubled with intermittent diarrhea and he was very prone to infection, with colds and chest infections almost every month. As well, his energy level was lower than what he felt was acceptable, making his work (in administration) an effort. As he explained: "I am tired all the time, even when I wake up." Clearly this was a condition that required careful evaluation in terms of helping his immune system to function more efficiently. It is not wise to try to boost the immune system where HIV is concerned, since there is evidence that aspects of the already depleted immune function are commonly overreacting in an effort to maintain control of the viral infection. Instead, a modulation of immune function is called for, using selected nutrients and herbs, along with an aggressive attempt at restoring bowel integrity using probiotic supplementation.

Frank's diet was tidied up somewhat according to the recommendations I provide in chapter 6, and a pattern of regular meals, smaller but more frequent, was instituted.

Over a period of eighteen months, a combination of supplementation with specific herbs and nutrients indicated for HIV-positive persons, along with probiotics (including *L. bulgaricus*) herbal antifungal treatment using echinacea, aloe vera, and a regular mouthwash and gargle (using a drop of tea tree oil in a tumbler of water as described in chapter 5); and a general approach to overgrowth of yeast in the bowels (which must be tackled if oral thrush is to be controlled) was found to keep the yeast to only a mild degree of activity in this man's mouth. His energy level increased, his ability to cope with stress was enhanced, and the frequency of recurrent infections was reduced to once or twice a year—a normal level. Seven years after his initial diagnosis, Frank continues to work and live a productive life with no obvious health problems apart from a mild degree of yeast activity in the mouth when he is excessively stressed at work. He has joined a support group, has regular massage supplied free by a leading AIDS charity in London, and practices relaxation, meditation, and yoga—and safe sex.

3. SUSAN, AGE THIRTY-NINE, AND ROBERT, AGE TWO MONTHS

Susan was in the early stages of pregnancy when I first saw her. She had a history of thrush going back many years, to her teens, when she had been prescribed antibiotics for acne. Subsequent episodes of cystitis, treated with more antibiotics, and a lengthy spell on the pill had reinforced the condition to the point where it was more or less permanent. The only variations were that from time to time it was even worse than the usual degree of irritation, discharge, and itching. Medical attention produced no more than short periods of relative ease, days rather than weeks, and she had virtually abandoned discussing her problem with her doctor. She consulted me because of her anxiety over the potential ill effects of yeast infection on her baby.

It is well known that during pregnancy yeast has an easier time making inroads because of hormonal changes, however, there are also limited options for treating candida during pregnancy because of the justifiable concern for the embryo's health. After careful evaluation of Susan's diet it was clear that she was excessively consuming sugar-rich foods, and this was modified in the process of prescribing a balanced and nutritious diet.

Supplementation with garlic and probiotics (acidophilus, bifidobacteria, and bulgaricus) is perfectly safe during pregnancy, and these were all suggested according to the guidelines outlined in chapter 5. I also suggested local applications of yogurt into which acidophilus powder was mixed, along with douching with aloe vera in water and the use of nondrug pessaries such as calendula. The objective was to contain the condition until natural controls could once again exert themselves after pregnancy. These tactics allowed Susan a more comfortable pregnancy and a safe delivery, after which time her yeast activity declined to a level that was significantly better than it had been before her pregnancy.

Unfortunately, within a few months of giving birth, her baby, Robert, was found to be suffering from both cradle cap—a yeast infection of the scalp—and diaper rash, and so he too was brought along for advice.

By keeping the baby dry (changing diapers more frequently than usual) as well as the frequent application of a talc that contained undecylenic acid, and a calendula cream and/or paste made from acidophilus and yogurt, the external manifestations of diaper rash were kept under control while internal probiotic methods were initiated.

The baby had regrettably not been able to be fully breast-fed by Susan due to very low levels of breast milk production and so a suitable probiotic for babies was prescribed (containing *Bifidobacteria infantis*), together with goat's milk, to supplement her limited milk production. It was suggested that fruit juices be provided rarely, and even then only in diluted form.

Cradle cap is a scaly skin problem that affects many newborns. It is a form of seborrhoeic dermatitis and often involves candida as well, especially if the symptoms include red bumps, pimples, or pustules. The various antifungal methods suggested for local application in chapter 5 usually control this problem: diluted tea tree oil, aloe vera juice, or acidophilus paste all help, as long as the internal imbalances are also being dealt with by means of a probiotic supplementation and a low-sugar diet.

The outcome for baby Robert was a happy one, with the diaper rash and cradle cap clear within two months.

4. EDDIE, AGE THIRTY-SIX

This young man was one of the first people I treated for candida as a major feature of his condition. He came to me after seven years of steadily declining health. His major symptoms (and there were many others) included bloating of the abdomen accompanied by nausea and flatulence, heartburn, and indigestion. His constipation had become chronic, and he exhibited a tendency to light-headedness and dizziness. He also experienced periodic attacks of shivering, followed by high temperature, all of which incapacitated him.

Prior to the onset of his condition his health had been good, but it started to decline suddenly after an attack of gastroenteritis while on holiday from his government job. He had been treated with a broad-spectrum antibiotic and described what happened afterward: "For the eighteen months following the gastroenteritis I suffered all the symptoms daily, which were so severe it resulted in my being unable to go to work for six months, and the remaining twelve months I went to work only with massive support from my colleagues, who shared my work load, and from understanding superiors, who allowed me to go home or rest when the attacks were severe."

When I saw Eddie he told me that there had been a gradual improvement in his condition during the years following the initial attack, until some twelve months prior to our first consultation, when after an acute attack he had experienced a return of all the original symptoms. He said, "At present I am struggling to cope with each day as it comes, and deal with this extremely debilitating and distressing illness as best I can."

In the intervening years between the onset of his illness and consulting me he had been seen by many medical practitioners. An endoscopy showed no disease of the bowel. He was checked for a malabsorption problem, and again no abnormality was discerned. He went to the Royal Homeopathic Hospital (London) on two occasions, and had also consulted an herbalist, an osteopath, and a medical specialist in allergies (a clinical ecologist). He had been placed on a rotation diet, which helped him to avoid repetitive contact with suspected food families, but which had little effect on his overall condition.

The time I first saw him his typical diet was as follows: Breakfast was *bacon* or *sausages* and tomato, rice cakes and *marmalade,* decaffeinated *coffee* and *fruit juice* (not fresh). Midmorning he ate some fresh *fruit.* Lunch was a salad and a baked potato plus *ham* or cottage cheese. The evening meal was either *chicken* or *pork* or *sausages* or fish, and vegetables. He had rice cakes and a hot *milk* drink before retiring. I have italicized those elements of his diet that are contraindicated in an anticandida diet (rice cakes are fine).

He appeared exhausted, but was a bright and intelligent man who I felt would cooperate actively in any program designed to assist his own recovery. After tests—including cytoxic tests to elicit specific foods to which he might be reacting, as well as hair analysis (low in chromium, iron, manganese, and selenium)—he was prescribed the following:

- An antiyeast, antifungus pattern of eating, low in carbohydrates
- Supplements of vitamins A, E, B_1, B_2, B_3, B_6, calcium pantothenate (B_5), calcium, magnesium, and manganese. Vitamin C was also added. The vitamin A was in emulsified form for easy absorption.
- A diet that included a seed and yogurt breakfast, a salad for lunch, and an evening meal of "safe" protein with vegetables.

At the time I saw Eddie the knowledge regarding biotin and acidophilus was not current, and the above program, which you will recognize as a modified version of that given in this book, had a remarkably good effect. Improvement began soon after the institution of the new program. Two months later, biotin and acidophilus were introduced. When I saw Eddie six months after the first visit, he had experienced at least a 50 percent improvement in all symptoms. There were still some days of exhaustion, but overall an upward trend in his health was noted, after seven years of steady decline. Confirmation of the involvement of candida came with an attempt early in the program to introduce an organic iron supplement, in a liquid, yeast-based form. This was met with an immediate return of constipation, which had more or less resolved itself. A check-up six months later found a continued improvement, with lapses in the diet producing confirmatory flare-ups.

By following an anticandida program, Eddie's condition continued to improve. Eighteen months after first seeing him he wrote to me to say, "Please accept apologies for my delay in contacting you. It is an indication of the progress we have made that I am well enough not to have to adhere to the program so strictly. I am very much better overall."

5. LIZ, AGE FIFTY

This patient consulted me with a history of extreme itching and inflammation of the skin of the neck and scalp over a period of a year. Liz had an earlier history of acne, which was treated (unsuccessfully) with antibiotics. She suffered from flatulence and had a history of colitis and a delicate digestive system. She had consulted an herbalist, with little results, and a hypnotist, who taught her relaxation and helped her to stop scratching the affected areas. Yet the condition remained as before. At the time of the consultation I was not yet aware of the work of Dr. Truss on candida, and so my approach was to use a nutrient supplementation, based on her general clinical picture, a nutritional questionnaire, a hair analysis, and her current symptoms. Her dietary pattern was excellent (which, since this turned out to be a candida problem, had probably saved her from far wider infestation).

Liz was placed on the following supplements, each taken orally: emulsified vitamin A, 60,000 I.U.; zinc orotate, 200 mg; calcium and magnesium orotates, 1 g each; chromium orotate, 10 mg; selenium, 50 mcg; and evening primrose oil (vitamin F), 1 g. I also suggested that she take yeast tablets as a source of vitamin B. At this point she wrote to me (she lived a considerable distance from my practice) saying, "I am following your suggestions carefully, except for the brewer's yeast. Over the years I have tried a number of times to take it, but it creates gas and is most unpleasant."

This set off alarm bells, for I had just read the first of Dr. Truss's articles that week. I immediately revised the diet, which, while good under normal conditions, nevertheless contained substances derived from yeast, and of course a certain amount of yeast-type food such as honey and muesli bars. After following this regimen, Liz cancelled her next appointment with me, saying that as her symptoms had disappeared, she felt the journey to see me was unnecessary. I quite agreed. A year later she remained symptom-free, including both skin and bowel conditions.

6. DINAH, AGE THIRTY-ONE

I was consulted by Dinah, a computer-programmer, with the following list of complaints: eyes bloodshot and irritated for the past nine months; odd aches in joints and muscles;

fingers slightly swollen; puffiness under the eyes (and some-times above) after sleep. Ten years prior to the onset of these symptoms she had had cosmetic surgery and diuretics, to no avail—her "eye-bags" remained unchanged. She had been on a macrobiotic diet as well, still with no improvement in her con-dition. Her periods were erratic and painful, and she reported that her breasts became swollen and sensitive at these times. She felt unnaturally tired a good deal of the time. There was a history in her family of bronchial problems and depression, from which she too suffered.

Dinah's typical diet consisted of the following: Breakfast was *store-bought muesli with added sugar* plus *milk* or *apple juice,* and once a week she had eggs and *bacon* and *sausage.* Lunch consisted of a cooked vegetarian savory dish or a *sand-wich.* Her evening meal included fish and rice, and occasion-ally some meat. During the day she had the odd *sweet* and had three cups of *tea* with *sugar,* plus *biscuits.* The italicized foods, as you can see, are not part of the anticandida diet outlined in chapter 6.

She had noticed a progressive inability to cope with alco-hol. Her diet was reformed to remove the sugars and milk, and to increase complex carbohydrates. She was prescribed (after appropriate tests) vitamin B complex, kelp (seaweed), evening primrose oil, vitamin B_2, glutamic acid (an amino acid), and the minerals chromium, iron, manganese, and selenium. Also prescribed were biotin and acidophilus, to be taken after meals.

Within two months, Dinah reported that her period had been on time for the first time in years, there had been less of a tendency to swell (eyes or breasts), and she was able to cope with alcohol (although it was in fact proscribed from her diet, which raises the problem of patients complying with instructions—a major headache for practitioners). Three months later her condition was vastly improved, and her tiredness, bloodshot eyes, and aching muscles and joints had all diminished to a point where they no longer bothered her. A year later she was symptom free.

7. ANDREW, AGE FORTY-NINE

Andrew was a recovering heroin addict and alcoholic, who had been clean and sober for eighteen months. He presented himself for advice and treatment with a long list of symptoms, including chronic fatigue, headaches, nausea, digestive distress (bloating, indigestion, intermittent diarrhea), skin irritation, itchy anus, and athlete's foot, as well as insomnia, muscular and joint pain, and anxiety and panic attacks. He reported that he had been sent to the hospital for his symptoms and had been given a diagnosis of moderate cirrhosis of the liver as well as a hepatitis C infection. The joint and muscle pain that Andrew experienced was, he reported, "like having the flu all the time," something that would define one of the main symptoms of fibromyalgia.

Andrew was already receiving regular acupuncture and reflexology treatments, as well as counseling via a support group accessed through social services. He felt that these were all helpful, particularly—although only temporarily—for his pain and fatigue symptoms. He had been referred to me by his doctor for nutritional and herbal advice in the hope that his digestion would be improved, despite already having seen a dietitian who had directed him toward a more balanced eating pattern in which his sugar intake had been severely cut. He was, he said, trying to stick to the new high-protein, high–complex carbohydrate (such as vegetables and whole grains) and low–simple carbohydrate diet. When he followed this advice, he noticed that many of his symptoms were indeed eased, but the bloating, diarrhea, itching, and fatigue remained almost daily occurrences.

A careful look at his medical history revealed that Andrew had had multiple antibiotic courses over the past twenty years, during which time his diet had been very poor, with simple carbohydrates as his main food source (sugars, fats, and, of course, alcohol). He was aware that his digestive symptoms were aggravated when he consumed sugary foods.

Yeast overgrowth (candida) was clearly a part of his complicated medical condition, and after some discussion he agreed that we should focus on three strategies:

1. Improve the ecology of his digestive tract to remove as much stress as possible on his already damaged liver and to encourage an improved nutritional status. As part of this process, a gentle detoxification program was to be followed, including both liver support and anticandida protocols.

2. A program of graduated exercise (toning, stretching, and aerobic) as well as breathing retraining would be followed, to gradually regain a degree of physical fitness. Emotional support would be encouraged alongside the counseling he was already receiving in the form of relaxation and meditation exercises, particularly autogenic training.

3. A periodic mono-diet (a rice-only diet) was suggested for thirty-six hours every two weeks for three months (about two pounds of organic brown rice, cooked and eaten in small portions throughout the day, and not less than two

quarts of water daily) to enhance detoxification. A combination of dandelion extract, artichoke, and milk thistle (*Silybum marianum*) was recommended to support liver function, as well as reduced glutathione (100 mg daily).

Anticandida measures included the use of horopito together with a daily supplement of probiotic organisms, and prebiotic FOS (fructooligosaccharides)—8 g daily in divided doses. The mucous membrane of the digestive tract was allowed to heal by means of an herbal/nutrient combination containing L-glutamine, slippery elm, marshmallow, and licorice (*Glycyrrhiza glabra*), taken between meals.

General nutritional support was suggested with an advanced antioxidant formulation (vitamins A and C, selenium, L-cysteine, a multivitamin/mineral supplement, and biotin as well as magnesium for his muscle pain symptoms).

The general dietary advice was for a high-protein (low-fat), high-fiber (low-sugar) lacto-ovo vegetarian diet, which included abundant vegetables (cooked rather than raw for ease of digestion).

He was taught a calming breathing pattern to help reduce anxiety symptoms; the exercises were both described and demonstrated.

After a shaky start during the candida die-off, when his headaches and general malaise were worse for two weeks, a gradual but eventually marked degree of improvement emerged over a four-month period (with several brief, minor setbacks along the way). Andrew experienced better digestion, fewer headaches, less muscle and joint pain, enhanced sleep, reduced anxiety, and more energy. By the end of the third month he had no signs of athlete's foot or anal itching and reported that he felt "close to normal."

I asked him to repeat the rice detox (eating only rice for thirty-six hours) once a month indefinitely after he reported an enormous degree of energy enhancement and sense of well-being for several days after each of these mono-diet periods. He was also advised to continue the probiotic and prebiotic strategies and liver support, but the antifungal herbs were stopped after five months.

This was a case of a severely compromised person who diligently stuck to his program after years of self-neglect. His health had been permanently compromised, but his yeast-related conditions have been eliminated, and his general health has improved. His underlying liver condition remains the same and will require caution for the rest of his life.

8. CONNIE, AGE SIXTY-FIVE

This quiet, retired teacher had first consulted with me many years prior to her appointment. In a note before she came to see me she reminded me that "I first saw you fifteen or twenty years ago over thrush issues. It was very helpful. For the last ten months I have had a puffy skin area round two of my fingernails, and these are not growing normally. The antibiotics prescribed by my doctor made it much worse."

At our consultation she appeared very anxious. This background of stress, along with the fungal nails, were the focus of the advice I offered her in notes sent to her after the appointment. "I strongly urge you to be strict about sugars that you have been snacking on (Kit-Kats, biscuits, cake)," I wrote. "An alternative to your evening porridge might be a protein drink (whey protein is one option, as dairy foods seem to be well tolerated, or a spirulina or other algae powder)." In addition, I recommended the following:

1. Probiotics: I explained, "From any health-food store you can purchase FOS (fructooligosaccharides), a prebiotic that supports beneficial bacteria. It's a nonabsorbed, sweetish, powdered product (most usually derived from Jerusalem artichokes) that you sprinkle on food or drink with water. About 7 to 10 grams a day, i.e., a heaping tablespoon, would be ideal."

2. *Saccharomyces boulardii* (a strain of anticandida baker's yeast); one capsule daily, an hour after any meal.

3. VSL #3, a high-dosage probiotic cocktail (450 billion organisms per sachet); one sachet daily, in water, between meals. I advised her to expect some bloating at first when starting probiotics.

4. I also recommended a form of nutrient clay (bentonite) that is mineral-rich and acts to detoxify the gut. Dosage is a teaspoon of the powder daily, on food.

5. Local treatment for the fingernail area consists of applications of tea tree oil morning and evening.

In addition to these recommendations for supplementation, I wrote, "I think it is clear that your health would improve if stress factors were reduced. As we discussed, this involves two elements: reducing the stress load and enhancing resilience/functionality. It may be useful to understand that stress involves anything to which we need to adapt. This includes changes in our normal routines and practices, which also means that all treatments that alter one's routine involve the stress of adaptation." I told her that it was desirable to introduce lifestyle changes slowly, rather than trying to make a lot of changes all at once, which can overwhelm an already stretched system. I provided her with some notes on specific breathing and relaxation exercises as well, which we had discussed in our consultation.

I heard nothing more from this woman until fifteen months later, when I received an e-mail from her with this message: "I have perfect health now—thank you from the bottom of my heart for changing my life."

9. GIL, AGE TWENTY-NINE

The tragic progression of ill health in this young lady's case is a clear indictment of the failure of many health professionals to recognize candida when it is staring them in the face. Before our consultation, Gil wrote to me at length:

> I have been suffering from pelvic inflammatory disease (PID) for almost two years now. The problem started when I began to experience lower abdominal pain and felt generally unwell. I was, at the time, using the contraceptive IUD, which I had removed, believing this to be the cause of the pain. [Prior to this, it turned out, Gil had been using the contraceptive pill, and she had a history of recurrent thrush.] However, [removal of the coil] had no effect and the pain became worse. Unfortunately, my doctor did not diagnose PID, and I therefore received no treatment in the early stages of the disease. Eventually I had to go to the hospital, where the gynecologist diagnosed PID through a laparoscopy. At that time there

was some damage to the fallopian tubes and adhesions in the pelvic area. I was put on to antibiotics, and for a time the condition seemed to improve. After a short time, however, I began to experience further attacks, and had to take larger doses of antibiotics regularly, and strong painkillers for much of the time. At times the pain was incredibly intense. I was finally admitted to a women's hospital in London for another laparoscopy. They found that both fallopian tubes were blocked, and it sounded as though damage/adhesions in the pelvic area had progressed further. Despite this I was told that the pain I was complaining of was psychological, and though they would be prepared to do tube reconstruction for fertility purposes, there was nothing more they could do for me. I subsequently visited a specialist, who said that my symptoms and pain were classic PID, but there was nothing he could do to help either.

My menstrual cycle had now gone from four to six weeks. Apart from the pain, other symptoms were active nausea, upset stomach, dizziness, and slight temperature. I also became very depressed. I finally had surgery after consulting a leading gynecologist. This consisted of removal of the left fallopian tube and reconstruction of the right; separation of adhesions to tubes, ovaries, and uterus through microsurgery; presacral neurotomy (removal of nerve to uterus); and steroid treatment to prevent regrowth of adhesions.

After this all was well until about five months later, when symptoms began again. Although the pain was not as severe as before, tests showed that the infection was active again. I was put on heavy doses of antibiotics.

It did not clear up, and I am now in my sixth week of antibiotics. The specialist told me that there was nothing more they could do surgically, and that I may have the condition for the rest of my life and must learn to live with it. I have a very positive attitude toward getting better and find it very difficult to believe that there is nothing else I can do to beat this disease, or at least fight it more effectively.

Gil's history indicated that she had commenced on this sad slide to ill health at the age of twelve, when cystitis was first apparent, after which she began a thirteen-year history of vaginal thrush. Following our consultation she went on the basic anticandida program outlined in earlier chapters: a high-fiber, low–refined carbohydrate diet, with no fungal foods; and supplements of biotin, acidophilus, olive oil, zinc, vitamin F, and garlic.

Two months later Gil reported that she was feeling quite a bit better, apart from a couple of bad spells from which she recovered more quickly than usual. About a year after starting the anticandida program, she wrote to me: "I have been feeling considerably better. The pain is now limited to a few days a month (around the time of my period). After my last laparoscopy the specialist said that it was the best result from that type of operation that he'd ever had. My remaining fallopian tube was tested and is clear, so I am a lot happier."

This is a clear and dramatic example of the tragedy that can occur when candida gets out of control in a young body— and demonstrates the effectiveness of the natural program outlined in this book.

10. SALLY, AGE THIRTY-FIVE

Sally was an actress who suffered from a continuous form of facial acne that was both unsightly and a huge disadvantage in her work, as well as being psychologically upsetting. This condition had been present since the age of fourteen. Her history was unremarkable apart from a highly stressful lifestyle, one surgery (cryosurgery) to deal with a cervical erosion, and a tendency to not ovulate regularly. In the past when under stress her skin would erupt into very large pustules.

Sally started on the basic anticandida program outlined in this book. Her protocol included a home-mixed seed, oatmeal, and yogurt breakfast, a salad-based lunch, and an evening meal of fresh organic protein and vegetables. She took pre- and probiotics along with supplements selected to enhance skin function—zinc, non-yeast-based B vitamins, Omega-3 capsules (from safe fish sources and flax seed), and the amino acid glutathione peroxidase. After just three months her skin regained its normal healthy appearance and she started ovulating regularly.

CONCLUSIONS

Candida is one of the least understood, most widespread causes of ill health in our midst. Precisely because it is known to be everywhere in the human body, this common yeast is largely ignored and not even considered when conditions such as that of Gil (with PID) is diagnosed. In the many cases cited by Dr. Truss, the details are similar to those described above. To this catalog of ills Dr. Truss has dealt with people who have been diagnosed with schizophrenia, manic depression, and multiple sclerosis. All of these sufferers were restored to good health with the application of the sort of program we have been considering, although Dr. Truss's program included an anticandida drug treatment (such as nystatin) as well.

A wider awareness of the diagnosis of candida could perhaps lead to a marked reduction in human suffering. Candida is not just a minor health irritant. It can destroy the physical and mental cohesion of a person in a very short period of time.

Preventing the spread of candida is accomplished by the same method as for treating an overgrowth of the yeast. The knowledge that we now have as to what makes candida spread is easy to understand and, fortunately, easily remedied by practical, natural methods. Let us hope that with the advent of modern Internet communication and the ease with which information can now be disseminated, knowledge about candida will become widespread among all health care practitioners.

Further Reading

In addition to the sources mentioned in the literature sections at the end of each chapter, the following sources are recommended:

DIET

Bohner, Sandra. *Sugar Free and Easy Candida Diet Recipes (Book 1): 20 Minute Meals to Heal Bloating and Yeast Infections.* CreateSpace, 2014.

Brostoff, Jonathan, and Linda Gamlin. *Food Allergies and Food Intolerance: The Complete Guide to Their Identification and Treatment.* Rochester, Vt.: Healing Arts Press, 2000.

D'Adamo, Peter, and Catherine Whitney. *Eat Right for 4 Your Type: Complete Blood Type Encyclopedia.* New York: Riverhead Books, 2002.

Dumke, Nicolette M. *The Ultimate Food Allergy Cookbook and Survival Guide.* Louisville, Colo.: AllergyAdapt, 2006.

Gedgaudas, Nora T. *Primal Body, Primal Mind: Beyond the Paleo Diet for Total Health and a Longer Life.* Rochester, Vt.: Healing Arts Press, 2011.

Halstead, Pauli. *Primal Cuisine: Cooking for the Paleo Diet.* Rochester, Vt.: Healing Arts Press, 2013.

Johari, Harish. *Ayurvedic Healing Cuisine: 200 Vegetarian Recipes for Health, Balance, and Longevity.* Rochester, Vt.: Healing Arts Press, 2000.

Malterre, Tom, and Alissa Segersten. *The Elimination Diet:*

Discover the Foods That Are Making You Sick and Tired—and Feel Better Fast. New York: Grand Central Life and Style, 2015.

Schmid, Ron. *Primal Nutrition: Paleolithic and Ancestral Diets for Optimal Health.* 5th ed. Rochester, Vt.: Healing Arts Press, 2015.

Vasey, Christopher. *The Acid-Alkaline Diet for Optimum Health: Restore Your Health by Creating pH Balance in Your Diet.* Rev. 2nd ed. Rochester, Vt.: Healing Arts Press, 2006.

Wagman, Gary. *Your Yin Yang Body Type: The Korean Tradition of Sasang Medicine.* Rochester, Vt.: Healing Arts Press, 2015.

Williams, Roger. *Biochemical Individuality.* Austin: University of Texas Press, 1998.

HEALTH

Bland, Jeffrey, and Mark Hyam. *The Disease Delusion: Conquering the Causes of Chronic Illness for a Healthier, Longer, and Happier Life.* New York: HarperWave, 2014.

Cooper, Celeste, and Jeffrey Miller. *Integrative Therapies for Fibromyalgia, Chronic Fatigue Syndrome, and Myofascial Pain.* Rochester, Vt.: Healing Arts Press, 2010.

STRESS

Sood, Amit, and the Mayo Clinic. *Mayo Clinic Guide to Stress-Free Living.* Cambridge, Mass.: Da Capo Press, 2013.

Online Resources

Author's note: A listing here does not mean recommendation. This section is for informational purposes only.

CANDIDA INFORMATION AND TESTING SOURCES

www.nationalcandidacenter.com/

www.betterhealthusa.com/public/156.cfm

www.creative-diagnostics.com/

www.gdx.net/product/yeast-culture-test-stool

www.greatplainslaboratory.com/home/eng/food_allergy_igg.asp

Index

BOOKS OF RELATED INTEREST

Amino Acids in Therapy
A Guide to the Therapeutic Application of Protein Constituents
by Leon Chaitow, D.O., N.D.

The Acupuncture Treatment of Pain
Safe and Effective Methods for Using Acupuncture
in Pain Relief
by Leon Chaitow, D.O., N.D.

Soft-Tissue Manipulation
A Practitioner's Guide to the Diagnosis and Treatment of
Soft-Tissue Dysfunction and Reflex Activity
by Leon Chaitow, D.O., N.D.

The Acid–Alkaline Diet for Optimum Health
Restore Your Health by Creating pH Balance in Your Diet
by Christopher Vasey, N.D.

Natural Remedies for Inflammation
by Christopher Vasey, N.D.

The Oil Pulling Miracle
Detoxify Simply and Effectively
by Birgit Frohn

Primal Body, Primal Mind
Beyond the Paleo Diet for Total Health and a Longer Life
by Nora T. Gedgaudas, CNS, NTP, BCHN

Colloidal Silver
The Natural Antibiotic
by Werner Kühni and Walter von Holst

INNER TRADITIONS • BEAR & COMPANY
P.O. Box 388, Rochester, VT 05767
1-800-246-8648 • www.InnerTraditions.com

Or contact your local bookseller